T0213812

Penile Carcinoma

Philippe E. Spiess • Andrea Necchi
Editors

Penile Carcinoma

Therapeutic Principles and Advances

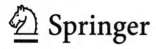 Springer

Editors
Philippe E. Spiess
Department of Genito-Urinary Oncology
Department of Tumor Biology
H. Lee Moffitt Cancer Center and
Research Institute
Tampa, FL
USA

Andrea Necchi
Vita-Salute San Raffaele University
IRCCS San Raffaele Hospital and
Scientific Institute
Milan
Italy

ISBN 978-3-030-82062-6   ISBN 978-3-030-82060-2   (eBook)
https://doi.org/10.1007/978-3-030-82060-2

This Springer imprint is published by the registered company Springer Nature Switzerland AG
The registered company address is: Gewerbestrasse 11, 6330 Cham, Switzerland

Foreword

I wish to congratulate Drs Andrea Necchi and Philippe Spiess and their colleagues who have authored this book, on this outstanding contribution to our knowledge relating to the contemporary management of those unfortunate patients who present with penile cancer. In contemporary medical practice it is essential that when dealing with rare medical conditions that we such pool our knowledge and resources and work collaboratively in a multidisciplinary team (MDT) setting. The development of reference centres is the only effective manner in which we can provide the optimal treatment of such conditions, thereby aiming for the best clinical outcomes for our patients. Over the last decade, this approach in such specialised centres has led to significant improvements in our understanding and management of penile cancer as a disease. This in turn has led to the implementation in reference centres to less invasive treatment with good outcomes in a number of patients with penile cancer, thereby avoiding unnecessarily radical surgery wherever possible. This clinical approach has proved very successful in the United Kingdom. It is with this in mind that the European Reference Networks (ERNs) on rare diseases were established. This allowed the European Association of Urology working closely with The European Commission to establish the eUROGEN network. Theses ERNs facilitate the confidential transfer of patient information to allow any clinician from across Europe to share their expertise, knowledge, and experience with others in an MDT setting, thereby facilitating the most effective management of patients with conditions such as penile cancer.

In this important reference work, the authors explore the ethos of this approach with a comprehensive review of the contemporary knowledge relating to penile cancer. They review the mechanisms of carcinogenesis and progression coupled with tumour pathophysiology and staging as a basis upon which to characterise tumours most effectively. Thereby, facilitating the individualisation of treatment based hopefully in the future on a more widely available genomic profiling of patients, which hopefully will provide dividends in the future. Clearly, in dealing with such a devastating condition, which is often disfiguring to the individual affected, with the consequent severe psychological impact on the patient and their partner, particularly where surgery is necessary.

Further chapters review the management of primary penile tumours with both penile-sparing and non-surgical approaches, partial and total penectomy, the management of inguinal and pelvic lymph nodes, and the difficult problem of bulky disease. The importance of an MDT approach is no more evident than when managing patients with neoadjuvant and adjuvant multimodal treatment for locally recurrent disease and metastatic disease.

Progress in most effectively treating penile cancer in the future can only be achieved by pooling the management of patients in reference centres. This will allow the evaluation of novel therapeutic approaches, both medical and surgical, and facilitate the development of clinical trials to provide an effective evidence basis upon which to recommend treatment.

The reader of this book will recognise the complexity of the management of this rare disease process. They should consider that as an individual clinician is unlikely to treat many patients with penile cancer during their career, they should reflect on the old dictum, "being a jack of all trades leads to potentially being a master of none". To obtain the best clinical outcomes for our patients with penile cancer, it is clearly inappropriate to manage them in isolation.

Christopher Chapple
Sheffield Teaching Hospitals NHS Foundation Trust
Sheffield, UK

Preface

Penile cancer remains a relatively infrequent malignancy cared for even at high volume centers across the world. In consequence, often patients can present in a delayed fashion often being unrecognized at an earlier stage of progression resulting in certain instances with dissemination to metastatic regional nodal or distant sites whereby imparting an adverse prognosis. Although both NCCN© and EAU© guidelines have established standards for optimal diagnosis and management of penile cancer patients, we know these guidelines are unfortunately not frequently adhered to, which highlights the critical necessity of not only enhancing educational resources for clinicians and healthcare team members but insuring patients and their families are aware that effective and often less debilitating treatment options may be available. Recent societies dedicated to advancing the care of infrequent genitourinary malignancies have been founded, including the Global Society of Rare GU Tumors™, which has as its primary mission to not only educate and promote patient advocacy for those impacted by these often under-represented tumors such as penile cancer but also promote and advance cutting-edge research in this arena through international collaboratives and sharing of educational resources throughout the global community, most notably in parts of the world were such resources may not be readily available.

In the present reference textbook, we will highlight meaningful advances that have been made in the fundamental understanding of the biological mechanisms of carcinogenesis for penile cancer by Dr. Maarten Albersen and colleagues from Leuven, Belgium. This will be followed by a part on the enhancements in penile cancer staging and key pathophysiologic concepts including a discussion on the emerging role of genomic profiling for penile cancer (in comparison to other squamous cell tumors at other distinct anatomic sites) by Dr. Jeff Ross and colleagues, which will provide a glimpse as to the emerging systemic therapies which maybe on the horizon. An important and often-not-talked-about consideration in managing penile cancer relates to the psychosocial impact of this often-devastating malignancy on patients and their families, which has been given its own dedicated part to raise awareness and provide the needed insight for healthcare professionals to provide a more holistic therapeutic approach to their patients and screen for potential depression and at times even suicidal ideation. Our reference book will then embark on a thoughtful discussion by international leaders on the current and emerging optimal treatment strategies to primary penile tumors, inguinal/pelvic lymph nodes, and locally recurrent disease. The importance of multi-disciplinary care in the management of advanced disease cannot be over-emphasized, and this will be highlighted in a part contributed to by Dr. Andrea Necchi and Dr. Peter Johnstone. Last but certainly not least, there are some exciting therapeutic avenues being explored to fundamentally re-define our treatment strategies to advanced penile cancer with many innovative approaches using a host of immunotherapeutic applications alone or in combination as well as the much anticipated International Penile Cancer Advanced (InPACT) trial, which is hoped to hopefully complete accrual within the next 2 to 3 years. Although many of these remain in the explorative phase in penile cancer research, they are being conducted as prospective trials often as basket trials along with other chemo-refractory squamous cell carcinomas originating from other anatomic sites such as the head and neck which will be discussed in our final part dedicated to an innovative clinical trials corner.

In conclusion, we would like to dedicate this book to our heroic patients and their families who have been unfortunately impacted by these devastating tumors but have steadfastly approached their diagnosis and treatment with unwavering courage and with an unyielding sense of hope. You truly inspire us all to not accept good or better as an acceptable treatment goal but rather increase our multitude of efforts to cure patients and provide them with the opportunities to live fulfilling and non-debilitated lives with their loved ones.

Tampa, FL, USA   Philippe E. Spiess
Milan, Italy   Andrea Necchi

Contents

Contributors

Mohamed E. Ahmed, MB, BCh Department of Urology, Mayo Clinic, Rochester, MN, USA

Maarten Albersen Department of Urology, University Hospitals Leuven, Leuven, Belgium

Hussain M. Alnajjar Institute of Andrology and UCL Male Genital Cancer Centre, University College London Hospitals NHS Foundation Trust, London, UK

Benjamin Ayres St. George's University Hospital, London, UK

Marco Bandini, MD Urological Research Institute, Vita-Salute San Raffaele University, Milan, Italy

Katherine Bobrek Department of Urology, Emory University, Atlanta, GA, USA

Gennady Bratslavsky, MD Department of Urology, Upstate Medical University, Syracuse, NY, USA

Sofia Canete-Portillo Department of Pathology, The University of Alabama at Birmingham (UAB), Birmingham, AL, USA

Jad Chahoud, MD, MPH Department of GU Oncology H. Lee Moffit Cancer Center, Tampa, FL, USA

Department of Medicine, University of South Florida, Tampa, FL, USA

Alcides Chaux Department of Scientific Research, Norte University, Asunción, Paraguay

Juan Chipollini Department of Urology, The University of Arizona, Tucson, AZ, USA

Laura Elst Department of Urology, University Hospitals Leuven, Leuven, Belgium

Joseph Jacob, MD Department of Urology, Upstate Medical University, Syracuse, NY, USA

Peter A. S. Johnstone, MD, FACR, FASTRO, FARS Departments of Radiation Oncology and Health Outcomes & Behavior, Moffitt Cancer Center, University of South Florida, Tampa, FL, USA

Vidhu B. Joshi, BSc Department of Urology, Mayo Clinic, Rochester, MN, USA

R. Jeffrey Karnes, MD Department of Urology, Mayo Clinic, Rochester, MN, USA

Grace Lee Rutgers Robert Wood Johnson Medical School, New Brunswick, NJ, USA

Viraj A. Master Department of Urology, Emory University, Atlanta, GA, USA
Winship Cancer Institute, Emory University, Atlanta, GA, USA

Bradley A. McGregor Lank Center for Genitourinary Oncology, Dana Farber Cancer Institute and Harvard Medical School, Boston, MA, USA

Asif Muneer Institute of Andrology and UCL Male Genital Cancer Centre, University College London Hospitals NHS Foundation Trust, London, UK
Division of Surgery and Interventional Science, University College London, London, UK
NIHR Biomedical Research Centre University College London Hospitals, London, UK

Reza Nabavizadeh Department of Urology, Emory University, Atlanta, GA, USA

Andrea Necchi, MD Vita-Salute San Raffaele University, IRCCS San Raffaele Hospital and Scientific Institute, Milan, Italy

George J. Netto Department of Pathology, The University of Alabama at Birmingham (UAB), Birmingham, AL, USA

Karl H. Pang Academic Urology Unit, University of Sheffield, Sheffield, UK
Section of Andrology, Pyrah Department of Urology, St James' Hospital, The Leeds Teaching Hospitals NHS Trust, Leeds, UK

Curtis A. Pettaway, MD Department of Urology, The University of Texas MD Anderson Cancer Center, Houston, TX, USA

Grant R. Pollock Department of Urology, The University of Arizona, Tucson, AZ, USA

Jeffrey S. Ross, MD Department of Urology, Upstate Medical University, Syracuse, NY, USA
Foundation Medicine, Cambridge, MA, USA

Malek Saad, BSc Lebanese American University, Beirut, Lebanon

Savan Shah, MD University of South Florida Morsani College of Medicine at H. Lee Moffitt Cancer Center, Tampa, FL, USA

Marta Skrodzka St. George's University Hospital, London, UK

Guru P. Sonpavde, MD Lank Center for Genitourinary Oncology, Dana Farber Cancer Institute and Harvard Medical School, Boston, MA, USA

Philippe E. Spiess, MD, MS, FRCS(C), FACS Department of Genito-Urinary Oncology, Department of Tumor Biology, H. Lee Moffitt Cancer Center and Research Institute, Tampa, FL, USA

Gigi Vos Department of Urology, University Hospitals Leuven, Leuven, Belgium

Nicholas Watkin St. George's University Hospital, London, UK

Alice Yu, MD, MPH Department of Genitourinary Oncology, Moffitt Cancer Center, Tampa, FL, USA

Jiping Zeng Department of Urology, The University of Arizona, Tucson, AZ, USA

Chapter 1
Mechanism of Carcinogenesis and Progression

Gigi Vos, Laura Elst, and Maarten Albersen

Introduction

Penile cancer is a rare cancer with a prevalence of 0.1–1 per 100,000 men in high-income countries. There is considerable variation in regional incidence depending on risk factors, such as human papillomavirus (HPV) infection, smoking, and poor hygiene, or protective factors, such as routine infant circumcision [1, 2]. Most penile cancers (95%) arise from the squamous cells of the glanular and preputial skin and are penile squamous cell carcinomas (PSCCs) [3]. Verrucous carcinoma, pseudo-glandular carcinoma, pseudohyperplastic carcinoma, adenosquamous carcinoma, and papillary squamous cell carcinomas are classified as non-HPV-related. Basaloid squamous cell carcinoma, papillary-basaloid carcinoma, warty(−basaloid) carcinoma, clear-cell carcinoma, and lymphoepithelioma-like carcinoma are HPV-related tumors [4]. There are two molecular pathways of carcinogenesis recognized by WHO: the HPV-dependent and the HPV-independent pathways [5]. A meta-analysis of global data showed that about half of PSCC are driven by HPV [2]. While the understanding of biological pathways and microenvironment in penile cancer is still limited, it is expanding and leading to the identification of possible therapeutic targets, which could significantly influence the prognosis of advanced penile cancer. Advances in genomic analysis in particular have provided transformative knowledge on the development and progression of penile cancer [6]. In this chapter, we will discuss mechanisms of carcinogenesis in PSCC.

G. Vos · L. Elst · M. Albersen (✉)
Department of Urology, University Hospitals Leuven, Leuven, Belgium
e-mail: laura.elst@student.kuleuven.be; maarten.albersen@uzleuven.be

P. E. Spiess, A. Necchi (eds.), *Penile Carcinoma*,
https://doi.org/10.1007/978-3-030-82060-2_1

1

Penile Intraepithelial Neoplasia

Penile intraepithelial neoplasia (PeIN) defines precancerous lesions, characterized by architectural and cytological abnormalities of the genital epithelium, which can further evolve into invasive PSCC. Again, PeIN is divided into two subtypes according to pathogenesis, undifferentiated (HPV-related) and differentiated (non-HPV-related) subtype, in analogy with invasive penile cancer [7]. Undifferentiated subtype lesions account for approximately 25% of the PeIN lesions [3, 4]. In addition, a classification of PeIN into three histologic grades has been implied (grade 1: mild dysplasia, grade 2: moderate dysplasia and grade 3: severe dysplasia) [3, 8]. However, this grading system is only applicable to undifferentiated PeIN, as differentiated PeIN is always classified as PeIN 3 [8]. A recent Dutch registry study in 380 patients found that 67% of lesions were PeIN 3 and progressed to a malignant phenotype in 7% of cases; PeIN 2 was found in 22% and progressed in 8%, and PeIN 1 was found in 11% and progressed to malignancy in only 2% [3, 8].

HPV-Dependent Pathway (Fig. 1.1)

HPV infection is an important risk factor in the development of penile cancer. A recent meta-analysis found, in a total of 4199 patients, that 50.8% (95% CI 44.8–56.7) of penile carcinomas are HPV-related [2]. There are over approximately 40 types of low-risk and high-risk HPVs known to infect the anogenital mucosa [4, 9]. The risk of infection increases with a previous history of genital warts and number of sexual partners [10]. HPV strains 16, 18, 31 and 33 have been strongly associated with penile cancer. It should be noted that low-risk HPVs are often found in penile cancer; nevertheless, they do not cause a significant dysregulation of RB or p53 [4].

HPVs are small, non-enveloped, circular double-stranded DNA viruses with an affinity for infecting basal cells of the epithelial mucosa via specific receptors such as heparan sulphate proteoglycans and $\alpha 6$ integrins, and physical micro-abrasions likely generated through sexual activity [3, 11]. The integration of HPV DNA into the host cell genome leads to the overexpression of viral oncoproteins (such as E6 and E7), initiating malignant transformation [4].

Oncoprotein E7 interacts with and inactivates the retinoblastoma tumor suppressor protein (pRB), resulting in the release of transcription factor E2F. DNA synthesis genes are activated, and the cell cycle becomes uncontrolled. In physiological circumstances, the release of E2F is facilitated by the pRB phosphorylation via cyclin D activity. This process is regulated by p16^{INK4A}. Due to the disturbance of the negative feedback via pRB, an overexpression of p16 INK4A can be observed [4]. Hence, p16INK4A may be used as a surrogate marker for the detection of active high-risk HPV infection in penile cancer [4, 12].

Oncoprotein E6 forms a complex with the tumor suppressor protein p53, causing the proteolytic degradation of p53, and inhibits BCL-2 homologous antagonist/killer (BAK) [3, 13, 14]. As a result, there is a disruption of DNA repair, growth arrest, and apoptosis. In addition, oncoprotein E6 supports cellular immortalization,

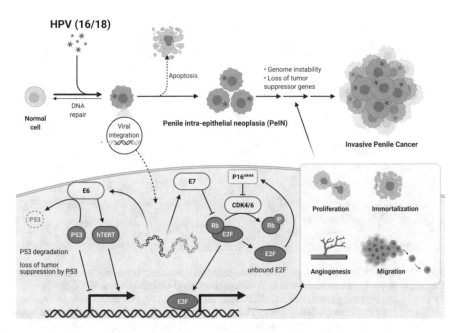

Fig. 1.1 The HPV-dependent pathway. The integration of HPV DNA into the host cell genome results in the overexpression of E6 and E7 oncoproteins. Oncoprotein E7 inactivates the retinoblastoma tumor suppressor protein (pRB), releasing transcription factor E2F. As DNA synthesis genes are activated, the cell cycle becomes uncontrolled. An overexpression of p16^{INK4A} can be found due to a disruption of the negative feedback via pRB. Oncoprotein E6 enables the proteolytic degradation of tumor suppressor protein p53, disturbing the process of DNA repair, growth arrest and apoptosis. Additionally, E6 may activate telomerase via c-myc-induced human telomerase reverse transcriptase (hTERT) expression, supporting cellular immortalization. (Figure created in Biorender)

by activating telomerase via c-myc-induced human telomerase reverse transcriptase (hTERT) expression [15].

Both oncoproteins, E6 and E7, interfere with the process of mitosis, inducing genomic instability [4].

The prognostic impact of HPV status remains unclear [16]. It has been suggested that the viral infection in HPV-related tumors leads to an increased immune reaction and a more favorable profile, resulting in a less aggressive form [17].

HPV-Independent Pathway (Fig. 1.2)

HPV-independent PSCCs are usually associated with tumor maturation and keratinization. HPV-independent penile carcinogenesis is less clearly understood compared to the HPV-dependent molecular pathway. The underlying mechanism is thought to be multifactorial predominantly through the effects of chronic inflammation and somatic gene alterations [3, 4].

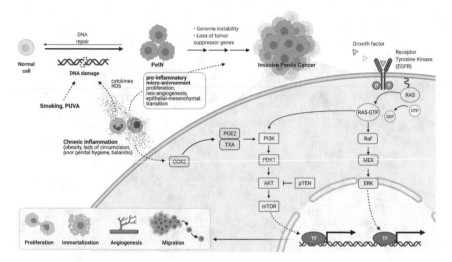

Fig. 1.2 The HPV-independent pathway Chronic inflammation and somatic gene alterations are thought to be the main mechanisms in HPV-independent penile carcinogenesis. DNA damage may be caused by smoking, psoralen-ultraviolet A light (PUVA) therapy, and reactive oxygen species (ROS) resulting from chronic inflammation. The cyclooxygenase-2 (COX-2) overexpression, initiated by chronic inflammation, induces an overproduction of prostaglandins (PGE2) and thromboxanes (TXA). Genomic alterations in mechanistic targets of the mTOR, tyrosine kinase pathways and DNA repair have been described. Some of these mutations can be targeted by currently available agents. Activation of the PI3K–AKT–mTOR pathway may also be linked to the activity of phosphorylated EGFR, leading to oncogenic and angiogenic processes. (Figure created in Biorender)

Recognized risk factors are related to the presence of chronic inflammation including lack of circumcision, phimosis, lichen sclerosus, obesity and inflammation; or direct mutagens such as smoking and previous UVA phototherapy [10, 18].

Chronic inflammation has an established role in the carcinogenesis of penile cancer. Cyclooxygenase-2 (COX-2) is an inflammation-induced enzyme found to be overexpressed in premalignant and malignant penile lesions [19]. The consequent overproduction of prostaglandins (mostly PGE$_2$) and thromboxanes leads to cell proliferation, invasion, and angiogenesis via various molecular pathways known to be involved in HPV-dependent carcinogenesis [4]. In mice, the knockdown of COX-2 has resulted in decreased tumor formation [20]. In addition, chronic inflammation can lead to direct DNA damage and genomic instability via the production of reactive oxygen species [21]. Furthermore, multiple somatic genetic alterations have been identified in the carcinogenesis of penile cancer, as a result of the advances in genetic sequencing. However, in penile cancer, the knowledge regarding DNA alterations and their association with cancer development remains limited.

Passenger mutations, in contrast to driver mutations, were believed to not have an important direct effect on the development and evolution of cancer. However, recent research findings suggest that an accumulation of these mutations may have role in carcinogenesis [6, 22–24]. In various studies, a number of carcinogenic driver genes were identified, such as RB1 overexpression, AR downregulation, BIRC5 overexpression were reported [6, 24]. BIRC5 encodes the survivin protein, which acts as an inhibitor of cell apoptosis [25]. Another recognized pathogenic driver is GPS1 tumor suppressor gene mutation [26]. The previously described tumor suppressor pathways (p16^{INK4A}/cyclin D/RB and p14ARF/MDM2/p53 pathways) also have a role in the HPV-independent cancer development [4]. The p16^{INK4A} gene can become inactivated by allelic loss or promotor hypermethylation [27]. This protein acts as a tumor suppressor as it blocks cell division by inhibiting cyclin D kinases 4 and 6. An association between the p16^{INK4A} inactivation or downregulation, and lymph node metastasis and disease recurrence has been described [27, 28]. In the evaluation of somatic genomic alterations, cancer tissue from 43 patients was analyzed. A panel that targeted 126 different genes was used, identifying TP53, CDKN2A, PIK3CA and HRAS as most frequently mutated genes [6, 29].

The tumor suppressor p53 plays an important role in protecting DNA from diverse insults through the regulation of cell-cycle checkpoints, DNA repair and apoptosis [14]. One study of 78 metastatic penile cancer patients found TP53 mutations and no HPV DNA in 73% of the sample [30]. It has been suggested that HPV-dependent mechanisms become gradually lost, with TP53 mutation becoming the main genetic mechanism driving metastatic progression in penile cancer [30]. Longitudinal studies will be required for the further investigation of this concept [6].

A number of cohort studies reported a link between the PI3K–AKT–mTOR pathway and the carcinogenesis of penile cancer, as they found an increase in immune-expression of mTOR and its stimulators (pEGFR, HER3 and HER4) [31, 32]. The overexpression of phosphorylated EGFR was associated with a HPV-negative status [6, 31]. It has been advocated that the high pEGFR detection results from E5 transcript-related EGFR activation and the absence of activation through the cyclin D/RB pathway by E6 and E7 proteins, which was shown to demolish the activity of E5 protein in HPV-infected cancer cells [6, 31, 33]. However, other study groups could not show this increased immune-expression. In order to detect the true role of the PI3K–AKT–mTOR pathway and its potential therapeutic significance, further research is necessary. Next to genetic alterations, it seems epigenetic changes (such as hypermethylation) and miRNA have a role as well in the carcinogenesis of penile cancer [6]. miRNAs are single-stranded, noncoding, small RNA fragments that act as posttranscriptional regulators of gene expression in several cancer types [34].

Tumor Microenvironment (Fig. 1.3)

Understanding the tumor microenvironment is crucial to understanding how and why some tumors remain indolent, whereas others are highly aggressive. A recent analysis by Ottenhof et al. indicated that HPV-positive tumors seem to have a higher propensity of tumor-infiltrating T cells with a stronger polarization towards T helper 1 cells and a more pronounced cytotoxic immune response and immune escape than

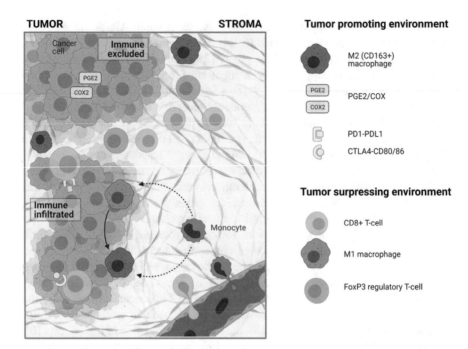

Fig. 1.3 Penile cancer microenvironment overview. The penile cancer microenvironment may be divided into tumor areas and stromal areas. Compounds like cyclooxygenase 2 (COX) enzymes and prostaglandin E_2 (PGE$_2$), with an immunosuppressive potency, contribute to the formation of an immune hostile tumor environment. The presence of M2 macrophages promotes angiogenesis and tumor cell migration. CD8+ T-cells, FoxP3+ Treg cells, and M1 macrophages have a role in tumor suppression. Cancer cells may evade the immune system, a process in which immune checkpoints, like programmed cell death-1 (PD-1)/programmed cell death ligand-1 (PD-L1) and cytotoxic T lymphocyte antigen 4 (CTLA-4), may have a role. (Figure created in Biorender)

HPV-negative tumors [35]. This represents a more mutated tumor type with higher T-cell inhibition properties. However, why these changes occur and their effects remain unclear. CD8+ T-cells and FoxP3+ Tregs have been described to be more prevalent in stromal areas than in tumor areas, in both HPV− and HPV+ tumors [35]. For CD8+ T-cells, increased infiltration in tumor areas, and thus a lower count in stromal areas, has been associated with lymph node metastases [6, 35, 36].

Tumor-associated macrophages (TAMs) include both the M1 macrophages, which have a tumor suppressor function, and the M2 macrophages, which are involved in tumor progression by creating an inflammatory environment that induces angiogenesis and tumor cell migration [35, 37]. Ottenhof and colleagues describe M2 polarization in intratumoral and stromal areas, and high intratumoral CD163+ macrophage infiltration in HPV-negative PSCC lymph node metastases [35].

COX-2 enzymes and PGE$_2$ are expressed in penile cancer tissue [38]. They have immunosuppressive potency and may contribute to the formation of an immune hostile tumor microenvironment. However, tumor cells can evade the immune system and its infiltrating cytotoxic CD8 T cells. Immune checkpoints, such as programmed cell death-1 (PD-1)/programmed cell death ligand-1 (PD-L1) and cytotoxic T lymphocyte antigen 4 (CTLA-4), may have a role in this process. PD-L1 expression is present in 40–60% of penile cancer patients [38]. Diffuse PD-L1 expression has been linked with a worse outcome, while tumor-stroma margin PD-L1 expression has been associated with a much better prognosis [35, 39–41]. This difference was suggested to be the result of marginal PD-L1 expression being induced by interferon γ, thus representing an active immune response, in contrast to diffuse PD-L1 expression which may be caused by genetic mutations [35]. Whether there is an association between PD-L1 expression and HPV status is still undetermined. Two studies observed no difference, whereas the Ottenhof et al. group found increased PD-L1 expression in HPV-negative cases (49% vs 32%, $p = 0.03$) [6, 35].

Conclusions

As a result of the advances in genomic analysis, our knowledge on the carcinogenesis of penile cancer is expanding. The subsequent identification of possible therapeutic targets could significantly influence the prognosis of advanced penile cancer.

Acknowledgments Maarten Albersen is holder of a research mandate for the Foundation against Cancer, Belgium.

References

1. Douglawi A, Masterson TA. Penile cancer epidemiology and risk factors: a contemporary review [Internet]. Curr Opin Urol. (Lippincott Williams and Wilkins); 2019 [cited 2021 Apr 25];29:145–9. Available from: https://pubmed.ncbi.nlm.nih.gov/30562185/.
2. Olesen TB, Sand FL, Rasmussen CL, Albieri V, Toft BG, Norrild B, et al. Prevalence of human papillomavirus DNA and p16 INK4a in penile cancer and penile intraepithelial neoplasia: a systematic review and meta-analysis. Lancet Oncol. 2019;20(1):145–58.
3. Thomas A, Necchi A, Muneer A, Tobias-Machado M, Tran ATH, Van Rompuy AS, et al. Penile cancer. Nat Rev Dis Prim [Internet]. 2021;7(1). Available from: https://doi.org/10.1038/s41572-021-00246-5.
4. Emmanuel A, Nettleton J, Watkin N, Berney DM. The molecular pathogenesis of penile carcinoma—current developments and understanding [Internet]. Virchows Archiv. (Springer Verlag); 2019 [cited 2021 Apr 1];475:397–405. Available from: https://pubmed.ncbi.nlm.nih.gov/31243533/.
5. Moch H, Cubilla AL, Humphrey PA, Reuter VE, Ulbright TM. The 2016 WHO classification of Tumours of the urinary system and male genital organs—Part A: renal, penile, and testicular tumours. Eur Urol [Internet] 2016;70(1):93–105. Available from: https://doi.org/10.1016/j.eururo.2016.02.029.
6. Aydin AM, Chahoud J, Adashek JJ, Azizi M, Magliocco A, Ross JS, et al. Understanding genomics and the immune environment of penile cancer to improve therapy. Nat Rev Urol [Internet] 2020;17(10):555–570. Available from: https://doi.org/10.1038/s41585-020-0359-z.

7. Diorio GJ, Giuliano AR. The role of human papilloma virus in penile carcinogenesis and Preneoplastic lesions: a potential target for vaccination and treatment strategies. Urol Clin North Am [Internet] 2016;43(4):419–425. Available from: https://doi.org/10.1016/j.ucl.2016.06.003.

8. Hoekstra RJ, Trip EJ, ten Kate FJW, Horenblas S, Lock MT. Penile intraepithelial neoplasia: nomenclature, incidence and progression to malignancy in the Netherlands. Int J Urol [Internet]. 2019 Mar 1 [cited 2021 Apr 1];26(3):353–7. Available from: https://pubmed.ncbi.nlm.nih.gov/30508877/.

9. Yugawa T, Kiyono T. Molecular mechanisms of cervical carcinogenesis by high-risk human papillomaviruses: novel functions of E6 and E7 oncoproteins. Rev Med Virol. 2009;19(2):97–113.

10. Thomas A, Vanthoor J, Vos G, Tsaur I, Albersen M. Risk factors and molecular characterization of penile cancer: impact on prognosis and potential targets for systemic therapy. Curr Opin Urol. 2020;30(2):202–7.

11. Yoon CS, Kim KD, Park SN, Cheong SW. α6 integrin is the main receptor of human papillomavirus type 16 VLP. Biochem Biophys Res Commun [Internet]. 2001 [cited 2021 Apr 1];283(3):668–73. Available from: https://pubmed.ncbi.nlm.nih.gov/11341777/.

12. Eich ML, del Carmen Rodriguez Pena M, Schwartz L, Granada CP, Rais-Bahrami S, Giannico G, et al. Morphology, p16, HPV, and outcomes in squamous cell carcinoma of the penis: a multi-institutional study. Hum Pathol [Internet]. 2020;96:79–86. Available from: https://doi.org/10.1016/j.humpath.2019.09.013.

13. Hoppe-Seyler K, Bossler F, Braun JA, Herrmann AL, Hoppe-Seyler F. The HPV E6/E7 oncogenes: key factors for viral carcinogenesis and therapeutic targets. Trends Microbiol. (Elsevier Ltd); 2018;26:158–168.

14. Hajiran A, Bracco T, Zemp L, Spiess PE. Leveraging innovative therapies with an evolving understanding of the molecular pathogenesis of penile squamous cell carcinoma. Urol Oncol. 2020;S1078-1439(20)30294-5.

15. Klingelhutz AJ, Foster SA, McDougall JK. Telomerase activation by the E6 gene. Available from: https://pubmed.ncbi.nlm.nih.gov/8598912/.

16. Vanthoor J, Vos G, Albersen M. Penile cancer: potential target for immunotherapy? World J Urol [Internet]. 2020 [cited 2021 Apr 1]; Available from: https://pubmed.ncbi.nlm.nih.gov/33145666/.

17. Sand FL, Rasmussen CL, Frederiksen MH, Andersen KK, Kjaer SK. Prognostic significance of HPV and p16 status in men diagnosed with penile cancer: a systematic review and meta-analysis [Internet]. Cancer Epidemiol Biomarkers Prev. American Association for Cancer Research Inc.; 2018 [cited 2021 Apr 1]; 27:1123–32. Available from: https://pubmed.ncbi.nlm.nih.gov/29987099/.

18. Douglawi A, Masterson TA. Updates on the epidemiology and risk factors for penile cancer [Internet]. Translat Androl Urol. (AME Publishing Company); 2017 [cited 2021 Apr 1];6:785–90. Available from: https://pubmed.ncbi.nlm.nih.gov/29184774/.

19. De Paula AAP, Motta ED, Alencar RDC, Saddi VA, Da Silva RC, Caixeta GN, et al. The impact of cyclooxygenase-2 and vascular endothelial growth factor C immunoexpression on the prognosis of penile carcinoma. J Urol. 2012;187(1):134–40.

20. Markosyan N, Li J, Sun YH, Richman LP, Lin JH, Yan F, et al. Tumor cell-intrinsic EPHA2 suppresses antitumor immunity by regulating PTGS2 (COX-2). J Clin Invest [Internet]. 2019 Sep 3 [cited 2021 Apr 1];129(9):3594–609. Available from: https://doi.org/10.1172/JCI127755.

21. Khansari N, Shakiba Y, Mahmoudi M. Chronic inflammation and oxidative stress as a major cause of age- related diseases and cancer. Recent Pat Inflamm Allergy Drug Discov [Internet]. 2009 Jan 10 [cited 2021 Apr 1];3(1):73–80. Available from: https://pubmed.ncbi.nlm.nih.gov/19149749/.

22. Budzinska MA, Tu T, D'avigdo WMH, Mccaughan GW, Luciani F, Shackel NA. Accumulation of deleterious passenger mutations is associated with the progression of hepatocellular carci-

noma. PLoS One [Internet]. 2016 Sep 1 [cited 2021 Mar 31];11(9). Available from: https://pubmed.ncbi.nlm.nih.gov/27631787/.

23. Kryukov G V., Pennacchio LA, Sunyaev SR. Most rare missense alleles are deleterious in humans: implications for complex disease and association studies. Am J Hum Genet [Internet]. 2007 [cited 2021 Mar 31];80(4):727–39. Available from: https://pubmed.ncbi.nlm.nih.gov/17357078/.

24. Marchi FA, Martins DC, Barros-Filho MC, Kuasne H, Busso Lopes AF, Brentani H, et al. Multidimensional integrative analysis uncovers driver candidates and biomarkers in penile carcinoma. Sci Rep [Internet]. 2017 Dec 1 [cited 2021 Mar 31];7(1):1–11. Available from: www.nature.com/scientificreports/.

25. Voges Y, Michaelis M, Rothweiler F, Schaller T, Schneider C, Politt K, et al. Effects of YM155 on survivin levels and viability in neuroblastoma cells with acquired drug resistance. Cell Death Dis [Internet]. 2016 Oct 13 [cited 2021 Mar 31];7(10):e2410. Available from: www.nature.com/cddis.

26. Feber A, Worth DC, Chakravarthy A, De Winter P, Shah K, Arya M, et al. CSN1 somatic mutations in penile squamous cell carcinoma. Cancer Res [Internet]. 2016 Aug 15 [cited 2021 Mar 31];76(16):4720–7. Available from: https://pubmed.ncbi.nlm.nih.gov/27325650/.

27. Poetsch M, Hemmerich M, Kakies C, Kleist B, Wolf E, Vom Dorp F, et al. Alterations in the tumor suppressor gene p16 INK4A are associated with aggressive behavior of penile carcinomas. Virchows Arch [Internet]. 2011 Feb 18 [cited 2021 Apr 1];458(2):221–9. Available from: http://www.ensembl.

28. Afonso LA, Carestiato FN, Ornellas AA, Ornellas P, Rocha WM, Cordeiro TI, et al. Human papillomavirus, Epstein-Barr virus, and methylation status of p16ink4a in penile cancer. J Med Virol [Internet]. 2017 Oct 1 [cited 2021 Mar 31];89(10):1837–43. Available from: https://pubmed.ncbi.nlm.nih.gov/28403538/.

29. McDaniel AS, Hovelson DH, Cani AK, Liu CJ, Zhai Y, Zhang Y, et al. Genomic profiling of penile squamous cell carcinoma reveals new opportunities for targeted therapy. Cancer Res [Internet]. 2015 Dec 15 [cited 2021 Apr 1];75(24):5219–27. Available from: https://pubmed.ncbi.nlm.nih.gov/26670561/.

30. Jacob JM, Ferry EK, Gay LM, Elvin JA, Vergilio JA, Ramkissoon S, et al. Comparative genomic profiling of refractory and metastatic penile and nonpenile cutaneous squamous cell carcinoma: Implications for selection of systemic therapy. J Urol [Internet]. 2019 Mar 1 [cited 2021 Mar 31];201(3):541–8. Available from: https://pubmed.ncbi.nlm.nih.gov/30291913/.

31. Stankiewicz E, Prowse DM, Ng M, Cuzick J, Mesher D, Hiscock F, et al. Alternative HER/PTEN/Akt pathway activation in HPV positive and negative penile carcinomas. PLoS One [Internet]. 2011 [cited 2021 Mar 31];6(3). Available from: https://pubmed.ncbi.nlm.nih.gov/21407808/.

32. Ferrandiz-Pulido C, Masferrer E, Toll A, Hernandez-Losa J, Mojal S, Pujol RM, et al. MTOR signaling pathway in penile squamous cell carcinoma: pmTOR and peIF4E over expression correlate with aggressive tumor behavior. J Urol [Internet]. 2013 [cited 2021 Mar 31];190(6):2288–95. Available from: https://pubmed.ncbi.nlm.nih.gov/23764082/.

33. Häfner N, Driesch C, Gajda M, Jansen L, Kirchmayr R, Runnebaum IB, et al. Integration of the HPV16 genome does not invariably result in high levels of viral oncogene transcripts. Oncogene [Internet]. 2008 Mar 6 [cited 2021 Mar 31];27(11):1610–7. Available from: https://pubmed.ncbi.nlm.nih.gov/17828299/.

34. Lu J, Getz G, Miska EA, Alvarez-Saavedra E, Lamb J, Peck D, et al. MicroRNA expression profiles classify human cancers. Nature [Internet]. 2005 Jun 9 [cited 2021 Mar 31];435(7043):834–8. Available from: https://pubmed.ncbi.nlm.nih.gov/15944708/.

35. Ottenhof SR, Djajadiningrat RS, Thygesen HH, Jakobs PJ, Józwiak K, Heeren AM, et al. The prognostic value of immune factors in the tumor microenvironment of penile squamous cell carcinoma. Front Immunol [Internet]. 2018 Jun 11 [cited 2021 Apr 1];9(Jun). Available from: https://pubmed.ncbi.nlm.nih.gov/29942303/.

36. Gooden MJM, De Bock GH, Leffers N, Daemen T, Nijman HW. The prognostic influence of tumour-infiltrating lymphocytes in cancer: a systematic review with meta-analysis [Internet]. Br J Cancer; 2011 [cited 2021 Apr 1];105:93–103. Available from: https://pubmed.ncbi.nlm.nih.gov/21629244/.
37. Qian BZ, Pollard JW. Macrophage diversity enhances tumor progression and metastasis. Cell. (Elsevier B.V.); 2010;141:39–51.
38. Stoehr R, Wendler O, Giedl J, Gaisa NT, Richter G, Campean V, et al. No evidence of microsatellite instability and loss of mismatch-repair-protein expression in squamous cell carcinoma of the penis. Pathobiology [Internet]. 2019 Jun 1 [cited 2021 Mar 31];86(2–3):145–51. Available from: https://pubmed.ncbi.nlm.nih.gov/30650417/.
39. Taube JM, Young GD, McMiller TL, Chen S, Salas JT, Pritchard TS, et al. Differential expression of immune-regulatory genes associated with PD-L1 display in melanoma: implications for PD-1 pathway blockade. Clin Cancer Res [Internet]. 2015 Sep 1 [cited 2021 Apr 25];21(17):3969–76. Available from: https://pubmed.ncbi.nlm.nih.gov/25944800/.
40. Howitt BE, Sun HH, Roemer MGM, Kelley A, Chapuy B, Aviki E, et al. Genetic basis for PD-L1 expression in squamous cell carcinomas of the cervix and vulva. JAMA Oncol [Internet]. 2016 Apr 1 [cited 2021 Apr 25];2(4):518–22. Available from: https://pubmed.ncbi.nlm.nih.gov/26913631/.
41. Garcia-Diaz A, Shin DS, Moreno BH, Saco J, Escuin-Ordinas H, Rodriguez GA, et al. Interferon receptor signaling pathways regulating PD-L1 and PD-L2 expression. Cell Rep [Internet]. 2017 May 9 [cited 2021 Apr 25];19(6):1189–201. Available from: https://www.sciencedirect.com/science/article/pii/S2211124717305259?via%3Dihub.

Part I
Tumor Pathophysiology and Staging

Chapter 2
Pathologic Features of Invasive Penile Carcinomas and Precursor Lesions

Alcides Chaux, Sofia Canete-Portillo, and George J. Netto

Introduction

Penile cancer is rare in certain geographical regions, such as the United States, Europe, Israel, and Japan, but highly prevalent in others, particularly in South America, Africa, and some regions of Asia [1]. The mean age of patients is 58 years, with most patients in their fifties to seventies [2]. The disease is sporadically seen in young adults.

Known risk factors include HPV infection, phimosis, cigarette smoking, and lichen sclerosus [3]. The previous history of penile tears, abrasions, or injuries is also associated with a higher risk of penile cancer, together with chronic balanitis and genital warts. Other risk factors include immunosuppression, human immuno-deficiency virus infection, treatment with psoralen and ultraviolet A, radiation therapy, and some other conditions such as lichen planus.

Most penile carcinomas are squamous cell carcinomas arising from the glans, coronal sulcus, or inner foreskin. The glans is the preferred site of origin, followed by the foreskin and coronal sulcus. Carcinomas originating in the shaft or the outer foreskin are rare.

A. Chaux
Department of Scientific Research, Norte University, Asunción, Paraguay
e-mail: alcideschaux@uninorte.edu.py

S. Canete-Portillo · G. J. Netto (✉)
Department of Pathology, The University of Alabama at Birmingham (UAB), Birmingham, AL, USA
e-mail: scaneteportillo@uabmc.edu; gnetto@uabmc.edu

© The Author(s), under exclusive license to Springer Nature Switzerland AG 2021   13
P. E. Spiess, A. Necchi (eds.), *Penile Carcinoma*,
https://doi.org/10.1007/978-3-030-82060-2_2

Precursor and Abnormal Epithelial Lesions

Penile Intraepithelial Neoplasia

Penile intraepithelial neoplasia (PeIN) references any degree of atypia and abnormal maturation in the squamous epithelium lining the glans, coronal sulcus, or foreskin [4]. Cytologic abnormalities can be subtle or affect most or the entire epithelial thickness. In all cases, extension beyond the basal lamina is absent. PeIN has been classified in PeIN I, II, or III or low and high-grade PeIN. "Erythroplasia of Queyrat" and "Bowen's disease" designations have been also used, adding confusion to the topic. These terms are best avoided and replaced by a consistent nomenclature.

PeIN includes differentiated, warty, basaloid, and warty-basaloid subtypes. Clinicopathologic features are distinctive among these subtypes. Foci of PeIN are found in association with penile carcinomas, either merging with the invasive component or adjacent to it. PeIN is also detected as single lesion during examination for other conditions.

When not associated with invasive penile carcinoma, differentiated PeIN tends to be localized in the foreskin of older males, while the other subtypes are preferentially located in the glans. However, it can affect any anatomical compartment. As single lesions, warty and basaloid PeINs are more frequently observed than differentiated PeIN, although when an invasive component is present the latter is more prevalent. Affected patients are younger than those with differentiated PeIN.

Macroscopically, differentiated PeIN presents as a single tan-white macula, plaque, or slightly raised geographical lesion. Warty and basaloid PeINs are grossly more variable, presenting as white, brown, or erythematous macules, plaques, or papules with a granular or velvety surface.

Microscopically, differentiated PeIN shows hyperkeratosis, parakeratosis, hypergranulosis, acanthosis, and elongated rete ridges with abnormal maturation and atypia. Atypia includes nuclear pleomorphism, coarse chromatin, and conspicuous nucleoli. These changes affect either a part or the entire epithelium. Differentiated PeIN can be also associated with lichen sclerosus.

In basaloid PeIN, the epithelium is replaced by a monotonous population of small-to-intermediate size cells with scant basophilic cytoplasm. Apoptosis and mitoses are common. In some cases, parakeratosis and isolated koilocytes are encountered. The surface is usually flat, but on occasions, one may observe a papillary growth pattern.

In warty PeIN, the surface shows a characteristic spiky aspect, with conspicuous koilocytosis and atypical parakeratosis. Cellular pleomorphism is more evident than in basaloid PeIN. In some cases, a mixed warty-basaloid PeIN is observed. Both components can be found in different adjacent areas of the same lesion or can form a superimposed pattern in which the upper third of the epithelium shows warty features while in the lower half the basaloid component predominates. A mixed differentiated-undifferentiated PeIN is also occasionally observed.

Differentiated PeIN tends to be associated with HPV-unrelated keratinizing variants of penile carcinoma such as usual, papillary, and verrucous SCC, while undifferentiated PeIN is mostly found with HPV-related tumors such as warty and basaloid carcinomas. When the PeIN pattern is mixed, the invasive component habitually shows mixed features.

Differentiated PeIN should be distinguished from squamous hyperplasia. The presence of epithelial maturation and the absence of cytological atypia are indicative of a hyperplasic process. Parakeratosis is a constant feature of differentiated PeIN and very rare or inconspicuous in squamous hyperplasia. Immunohistochemistry for p53 and Ki-67 can aid in the differential diagnosis [5].

Basaloid PeIN should be distinguished from urothelial carcinoma in situ of the distal urethra. Immunohistochemical markers of urothelial lineage, such as uroplakin-III, thrombomodulin, and GATA3 and cytokeratins 7 and 20, are helpful in difficult cases [6]. Overexpression of p16INK4a is characteristic of basaloid PeIN but may also be presenting urothelial carcinomas [7]. Warty PeIN can be confused with condyloma acuminatum. The presence of cytological atypia and the identification of high-risk HPV (16 and 18) are indicative of PeIN. Overexpression of p16INK4a, consistently absent in condylomata, can also be helpful.

Lichen Sclerosus

Previously known as balanitis xerotica obliterans, lichen sclerosus is a chronic inflammatory and sclerotic condition affecting the penis and vulva [8]. Its frequent association with differentiated PeIN and SCC subtypes, especially HPV-unrelated, indicates a precancerous role [9]. The etiology is unknown but several conditions, such as autoimmune diseases and immunologic dysregulations, are associated with this disease. Lichen sclerosus has been associated with the presence of HLA DQ7 haplotype as well as DR7, DQ8, DQ9, and DR4.

Lichen sclerosus has a predilection for the foreskin and glans. It manifests as irregular whitish atrophic areas located in the foreskin or perimeatal area. Some degree of phimosis is common. In advanced cases, extensive sclerosis narrows the preputial ring. Squamous hyperplasia, differentiated PeIN, or even invasive SCC can be associated. Lichen sclerosus is often multicentric, may affect multiple anatomical compartments, and can even extend into the distal urethra.

Microscopically, lichen sclerosus is characterized by the presence of epithelial atrophy, vacuolar degeneration of the basal layer, and dense hyalinization of subepithelial tissues. A band-like lymphocytic infiltrate is common. Edema of the lamina propria is observed in some cases.

Atrophic areas can be intermingled with foci of squamous hyperplasia or differentiated PeIN. In the latter, the term "atypical lichen sclerosus" is appropriate. These atypical changes are more frequent when lichen sclerosus is found in the adjacent areas of invasive carcinoma.

Sometimes, the areas of hyalinization are scant, or the edematous changes are prominent, impeding the recognition of the lesion. Care should be taken to recognize subtle forms of differentiated PeIN since the malignant potential of typical and atypical lichen sclerosus is different.

Squamous Hyperplasia

Squamous hyperplasia implies a reactive thickening of the epithelium covering the glans, coronal sulcus, or foreskin. Squamous hyperplasia is often associated with areas of differentiated PeIN and lichen sclerosus or other dermatoses, suggesting a precancerous role [10, 11]. Squamous hyperplasia is more likely to be encountered in association with low-grade variants of squamous cell carcinomas such as usual, papillary, and verrucous carcinomas, than HPV-related tumors (basaloid and warty carcinomas) [11].

Macroscopically, the tan to white lesion has irregular borders, and at times, slightly raised and pearly appearance. Histologically, it is characterized by acanthosis and hyperkeratosis, orderly epithelial maturation, and lack of nuclear atypia. Parakeratosis is typically absent.

Four patterns of growth can be identified: flat, papillary, pseudoepitheliomatous, and verrucous. Squamous hyperplasia should be distinguished from differentiated PeIN and low-grade SCC variants. The presence of any degree of nuclear atypia, altered epithelial maturation, and parakeratosis should prompt the diagnosis of PeIN. Positivity for p53 and Ki-67 above the basal layer is indicative of intraepithelial squamous neoplasia. Invasive pseudohyperplastic carcinoma (see below) can be confused with squamous hyperplasia. However, in pseudohyperplastic carcinoma, the underlying epithelial nests are irregular in shape, peripheral nuclear palisading is inconspicuous, the stromal reaction is prominent, and nuclear atypia is present, albeit minimal.

Distinguishing verrucous carcinoma from verrucous squamous hyperplasia can sometimes be difficult. Here again, the presence of nuclear atypia and stromal reaction favors a neoplastic process. Clinically, verrucous carcinomas are larger, and more exophytic than squamous hyperplasia. Other verruciform tumors, such as papillary and warty carcinomas, can also enter the differential diagnosis. Marked papillomatosis, prominent fibrovascular cores, and koilocytosis favor a warty carcinoma. In papillary carcinoma, papillae are longer and fibrovascular cores are more prominent. In both carcinomas, nuclear atypia is present.

HPV-Unrelated Subtypes

Usual Squamous Cell Carcinoma

Macroscopically, tumors are exophytic, endophytic, or ulcerative, forming irregular white-gray nodules measuring from few millimeters to large (around 2–50 mm) neoplasms. Tumors tend to be larger in high-risk geographical areas [12, 13]. On cut surface, the tumor can be seen involving lamina propria, dartos, corpus spongiosum, or corpora cavernosa.

Microscopically, well-differentiated (grade 1, Fig. 2.1a) carcinomas are composed of large irregular squamous sheets and/or infiltrating nests. Central keratinization with pearl formation is frequent. In moderately differentiated (grade 2, Fig. 2.1b) squamous cell carcinoma, tumor nests are usually more irregular and smaller in size. Nuclear atypia is evident, and mitoses are identifiable. Poorly differentiated (grade 3, Fig. 2.1c) carcinomas consist of even smaller nests, cords, trabeculae, or isolated anaplastic cells. Keratinization is focal if any. Nuclear typia and mitoses are conspicuous. Histologic grade can be heterogenous within a given tumor. Stromal host reaction and chronic inflammatory infiltrate are present [14]. Squamous hyperplasia and differentiated PeIN are often encountered adjacent to invasive carcinoma [15]. Lichen sclerosus is present in up to half of the cases [8].

Biologic behavior is mainly related to histological grade, thickness/depth of invasion, and presence of perineural invasion. Local and regional recurrences, usually due to incomplete resection, are not exceptional and occur in one-third of the cases [12]. Inguinal lymph node metastases develop in up to 40% of patients with usual squamous cell carcinoma. Tumors with nodal involvement tend to be larger, thicker, of higher grade, and deeply invasive when compared with non-metastasizing squamous cell carcinoma. The mortality rate of usual squamous cell carcinoma ranges from 20% to 38%. The 10-year survival rate is 78% [12, 16].

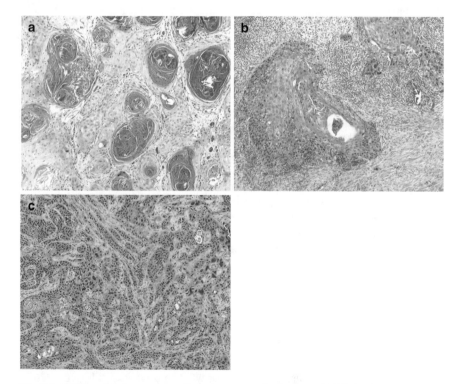

Fig. 2.1 HPV-unrelated squamous cell carcinoma, usual subtype: well-differentiated/grade 1 (**a**), moderately differentiated/grade 2, (**b**) and poorly differentiated/grade 3 (**c**)

Verrucous Carcinoma

Verrucous carcinomas are exophytic, verruciform, white-gray neoplasms. Most tumors are unicentric but multicentric cases are also found. Most are superficial but may occasionally involve the corpus spongiosum or preputial dartos. Involvement of corpus cavernosum is infrequent. The distinctive feature of this tumor is the sharp boundary between tumor and stroma, which can be observed better at the cut surface. Tumor invading erectile tissues maintain its broad base and expansive borders. Pure verrucous carcinomas do not metastasize, irrespective of their depth of invasion. If one observes foci of irregular invasion, usually of higher histological grade, the tumor should be then classified as usual-verrucous carcinoma (see below), which carries a different prognosis.

Microscopically, papillomatosis, hyperkeratosis, and acanthosis are typical. Papillae do not have a central fibrovascular core. Keratohyalin granules, parakeratosis, and vacuolated cells (lacking nuclear wrinkling and binucleation, distinct from the koilocytotic cells of warty carcinoma) are noted at the surface. Tumors are well-differentiated, with prominent intercellular bridges, and minimal or no nuclear atypia. The tumor base is broad, with pushing, regular, and expansive borders. Associated lesions are squamous hyperplasia (flat or verrucous), differentiated PeIN, and lichen sclerosus [8]. Immunohistochemistry for p16 and HPV are usually negative. Proliferation index is low on Ki67 stains [17–20].

Hybrid Verrucous Carcinoma

Verrucous carcinoma, as described above, can be admixed with usual squamous cell carcinoma [21]. Recognizing such hybrid tumors is important given the impact on outcome [22, 23]. Macroscopically, the cut surface is white, solid with an irregular to well-defined tumor front. Microscopically, in addition to verrucous carcinoma, we observe an irregular, destructive invasive front, corresponding to the usual squamous cell carcinoma component. Hybrid verrucous carcinomas are usually negative for HPV and p16. Hybrid verrucous carcinomas are considered higher-grade tumors that invade deeper into penile anatomical levels compared to pure verrucous carcinomas. They have the potential for nodal metastasis, tumor dissemination, and death. Inguinal metastases, usually absent in verrucous carcinoma, can occur in hybrid verrucous carcinomas [20].

Papillary Squamous Cell Carcinoma, Not Otherwise Specified (NOS)

Papillary NOS carcinomas are exophytic, verruciform tumors with hyperkeratosis and papillomatosis [24]. The cut surface is white with a serrated surface and a poorly delineated interface between tumor and stroma. More than half of these tumors invade up to corpus spongiosum or dartos.

Microscopically, papillary carcinomas are well-to-moderately differentiated. The papillae are complex, short or elongated, spiky or blunt, with or without a central fibrovascular core reaching the top. Koilocytosis is absent. The base of the lesion is jagged, with irregular nests of infiltrating squamous cell carcinoma. Most papillary carcinomas are negative for HPV and p16 [25, 26]. The prognosis is good. The recurrence rate is about 12%. The rate for inguinal lymph node metastases is low, ranging from 0% to 12%.The mortality rate ranges from 0% to 6% [12, 16].

Carcinoma Cuniculatum

Carcinoma cuniculatum corresponds to a complex, deeply penetrating, low-grade carcinoma with verrucous features and a burrowing growth pattern simulating rabbit holes [27, 28]. Multiple anatomical compartments are usually affected. Glans and coronal sulcus are usually involved. The cut surface reveals deep invaginations with narrow and elongated neoplastic sinus tracts connecting to the surface of the tumor. Extension to corpus spongiosum and corpus cavernosum is common. The boundaries between tumor and stroma remain sharply delineated.

Microscopically, hyperkeratosis, papillomatosis, and acanthosis are observed. The tumor cells are well-differentiated, and koilocytes are absent. The sinuses and cysts contain hyperkeratotic debris. Foci of squamous cell carcinoma with a destructive invasive pattern are sometimes found. HPV is negative [26]. Despite the deep penetration, inguinal involvement or systemic dissemination is unlikely [27, 29].

Pseudohyperplastic Carcinoma

Pseudohyperplastic carcinoma is a multicentric, low-grade carcinoma simulating pseudoepitheliomatous hyperplasia, mostly affecting the foreskin of older patients, and associated with lichen sclerosus [30]. The diagnosis can be challenging in small biopsies.

Macroscopically, tumors are flat or slightly elevated, white and granular. Microscopically, an orderly downward proliferation of nests is seen simulating pseudoepitheliomatous hyperplasia. The nests are composed of well-differentiated squamous cells with minimal atypia, surrounded by a reactive stroma. Tumors usually invade superficial levels, up to dartos in the foreskin and up to lamina propria in the glans. Separate or immediately adjacent foci of squamous hyperplasia, differentiated PeIN, and usual or verrucous squamous cell carcinomas are found in multicentric tumors. Immunohistochemistry for p16 and HPV is negative. The prognosis is excellent with no inguinal nodal metastases. Recurrence after circumcision may occur.

Sarcomatoid Carcinoma

Sarcomatoid carcinoma is an aggressive variant of penile carcinoma composed of spindle, pleomorphic, or polymorphic tumor cells at times admixed with foci of epithelioid cells with squamous features [31]. Sarcomatoid carcinomas arise de novo, or as a secondary sarcomatoid transformation of a recurrent usual squamous cell carcinoma, or following radiation therapy of a primary penile carcinoma [32]. Most tumors, due to their large size, affect multiple epithelial compartments, but the glans is the preferred site.

Macroscopically, sarcomatoid carcinomas are irregular, white-gray, or reddish hemorrhagic polypoid masses. The cut surface shows a dark reddish, necrotic, and hemorrhagic neoplasm with deep invasion into corpus spongiosum and corpora cavernosa. Microscopically, the spindle cells predominate, with interlacing bundles of atypical cells, resembling fibrosarcoma, leiomyosarcoma, fibrous histiocytoma, myxosarcoma, liposarcoma, hemangiopericytoma, angiosarcoma, or rhabdomyosarcoma [33–36]. Foci of osteosarcomatous and chondrosarcomatous differentiation are described. Giant cells may be prominent. Vascular and perineural invasion, as well as direct urethral invasion, are common findings. Necrosis is prominent, and mitoses are numerous. Immunohistochemical markers for sarcomatoid carcinomas include vimentin, p53, 34βE12, p63, EMA, AE1/AE3, and Cam 5.2, which are at least focally positive. It has been reported that muscle-specific actin, smooth muscle actin, desmin, and S-100 are negative in these tumors [31], although it is known that sarcomatoid carcinomas of other sites can be positive for SMA. Most cases are HPV negative [31, 37].

Sarcomatoid carcinoma is the most aggressive primary penile carcinoma. Patients may present with simultaneous nodal and systemic metastases. Inguinal nodal metastasis appears in up to 90% of the patients, and the mortality rate is 40%–75%. Local and systemic recurrences are common (two-thirds of cases), and most patients die within a year [38].

Pseudoglandular Carcinoma

Pseudoglandular carcinoma is characterized by acantholysis leading to the development of pseudoglandular or adenoid spaces [39]. Compared to the usual subtype, pseudoglandular carcinomas are higher grade, invade deeper anatomical structures, and are associated with a higher incidence of regional metastases and mortality.

Macroscopically, the tumors are large, irregular and white-gray in color invading into corpora spongiosa or cavernosa. The surface is ulcerative or exophytic. Microscopically, pseudoglandular features comprise 30% to 85% of the tumor, with a multicystic or honeycomb appearance at low magnification. The pseudoglandular spaces are lined by atypical flat, cubical, or cylindrical cells. The spaces are partially filled with an amorphous eosinophilic material containing keratin, acantholytic cells, and necrotic debris. Vascular and perineural invasions are frequent. Immunohistochemistry for p16 and HPV is usually negative.

Adenosquamous Carcinoma

Adenosquamous carcinomas are biphasic tumors composed of squamous and true glandular elements. The mucinous glandular component could be histogenically related to embryologically misplaced mucous cells occasionally found in the perimeatal squamous epithelium of the glans, goblet cells in the squamous epithelium of the foreskin, or aberrant differentiation of neoplastic squamous epithelium [40–43].

Macroscopically, adenosquamous carcinoma forms a granular, white-gray, firm nodules. The cut surface reveals an irregular tumor replacing most of the glans. Microscopically, the squamous cells usually predominate. The glands are lined by cubical or cylindrical epithelium and have intraluminal and intracellular mucin. Immunohistochemistry for CEA is positive in the glandular component. High molecular weight cytokeratin 34βE12 is positive in both components [40]. Local recurrence is observed in up to 25% of the patients [12]. Inguinal nodal metastasis ranges from 43% to 50%. However, the mortality rate is low, ranging from 0% to 14% [12, 38].

Mucoepidermoid Carcinoma

Mucoepidermoid carcinoma is a salivary-type neoplasm composed of an admixture of squamous cell with mucin-secreting cells in the form of intracellular mucin rather than true gland formation [44–46]. Macroscopically, mucoepidermoid carcinomas are irregular, ulcerated, white-gray masses affecting glans, and extending into the coronal sulcus or foreskin. The cut surface shows an infiltrating tumor extending to the corpus spongiosum. Microscopically, the tumor is moderately differentiated, with keratinizing squamous cell carcinoma intermingled with groups of mucin-secreting cells. Extracellular mucinous lakes may be present. There is no glandular differentiation. HPV is negative. Inguinal metastases are infrequent, and the prognosis is good.

HPV-Related Subtypes

Basaloid Carcinoma

Basaloid carcinoma is an HPV-related tumor [41]. The glans is the most frequent primary location. Macroscopically, the tumor presents as an ulcerated, irregular, solid mass. Microscopically, a downward proliferation of dense solid cellular nests separated by scant stroma is observed. The poorly differentiated squamous cells are small-to-intermediate size and basophilic with scant cytoplasm (Fig. 2.2a). Mitoses are numerous, and nucleoli are inconspicuous. At their centers, the tumor nests may contain necrotic cellular or keratin debris. Basaloid carcinomas tend to invade deep

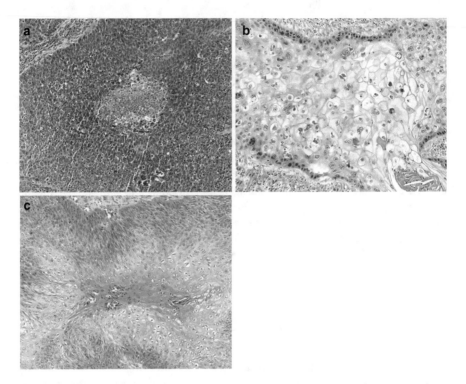

Fig. 2.2 HPV-related squamous cell carcinoma subtypes: (**a**) basaloid, (**b**) warty, and (**c**) warty-basaloid

erectile tissues. Vascular and perineural invasion are frequent findings. Basaloid carcinomas are usually positive for p16 and CK 34βE12. HPV-16 is the most found serotype [47]. On occasions, basaloid carcinomas can form papillae, simulating a papillary urothelial carcinoma [42].

Basaloid carcinoma is an aggressive neoplasm with a high incidence of nodal metastasis in most patients. Local recurrence is among the highest for penile squamous cell carcinoma when treated with organ-sparing surgery [13, 48]. Mortality rate is up to two-thirds of patients [1].

Warty Carcinoma

Warty carcinoma is an HPV-related, exophytic, cauliflower-like, verruciform tumor, usually affecting multiple anatomic compartments [49, 50]. Macroscopically, the tumor is white-gray in color with a granular texture. The cut surface shows a papillary neoplasm with condylomatous papillae. Microscopically, the condylomatous papillae are long and undulating with a central fibrovascular core and a jagged tumor front. The most conspicuous microscopic finding is the presence of koilocytes. In the koilocytes, the nuclei are enlarged in size, wrinkled, and hyper-chromatic, with frequent binucleation or multinucleation (Fig. 2.2b). Perinuclear clear halos and individual cell necrosis are common.

Invasion to erectile tissues is common. Vascular and perineural invasion are uncommon. Warty carcinomas are positive for p16 in more than half of the cases. Local recurrence after penectomy occurs in 10% of warty carcinomas and inguinal lymph node metastasis in about 17–18%. Systemic dissemination is rare and the mortality rate is low [12, 16, 49, 50].

Warty-Basaloid Carcinoma

Warty-basaloid carcinoma is an HPV-related tumor with mixed warty and basaloid features [51]. Macroscopically, tumors are white-gray large, irregular masses affect-ing multiple compartments. The cut surface is tan-to-white, solid, or mixed papil-lomatous on the surface and solid in deeper invasive areas. In most cases, the tumor deeply penetrates in the corpus spongiosum, dartos, or corpora cavernosa. Microscopically, the biphasic tumors have variable proportions of warty and basa-loid components. The most common pattern consists of a superficial warty compo-nent, with basaloid features in deep areas. Another pattern is characterized by the presence of tumor nests with central warty clear cells and peripheral basaloid cells (Fig. 2.2c). Vascular invasion is seen in one-half and perineural invasion in one-quarter of the cases. HPV is detected in most cases, either by PCR or by p16 immunohistochemistry.

Prognosis is intermediate between pure warty and basaloid carcinomas. Inguinal nodal metastases are present in about one-half of patients. About one-third of patients die from disseminated disease.

Medullary Carcinoma

Medullary carcinoma is a poorly differentiated carcinoma composed of anaplastic large cells with prominent nucleoli, associated with a rich inflammatory infiltrate [52]. Most primary tumors are located in the glans. Macroscopically, the tumors are large, irregular, white-gray masses destroying most of the glans and secondarily extending to the coronal sulcus and inner foreskin. Microscopically, the carcinoma cells are arranged in large sheets, solid nests, or trabeculae. Nuclei are large, pleo-morphic, with prominent eosinophilic nucleoli. Mitoses are abundant. HPV is detected in most cases.

Clinical and follow-up information of patients with medullary carcinoma is scant. However, their associated adverse pathological prognostic features, such as high histological grade and deep invasion of corpora cavernosa, suggest aggressive clinical behavior.

Clear Cell Carcinoma

Clear cell carcinomas are aggressive tumors growing in confluent sheets or nests composed of clear cells arising in the mucosal squamous epithelium of the penis [53]. Tumors preferentially involve the glans, with extension to coronal sulcus or foreskin. Macroscopically, clear cell carcinomas are large, white-gray, granular, irregular masses with ulceration of the glans epithelial surface. The cut surface shows a massive tumor invading erectile tissues. Microscopically, the solid nests of clear cells display central comedonecrosis. Nuclei are hyperchromatic, rounded, ovoid, or wrinkled. Binucleation is common. Inguinal nodal metastases are frequent and tumor dissemination is frequently seen. The mortality rate is high.

Lymphoepithelioma-like Carcinoma

Lymphoepithelioma-like carcinoma is a poorly differentiated tumor with loose cells obscured by a dense inflammatory infiltrate, resembling the lymphoepithelial-like carcinoma of the nasopharynx [54]. Macroscopically, the white-gray tumor mainly affects the glans. Microscopically, a "syncytial" growth pattern is imparted by the irregular sheets, nests and trabeculae within a dense lymphoplasmacytic and eosinophilic infiltrate, which obscures tumor cell boundaries. Immunohistochemistry for p63 is useful for the identification of epithelial cells. Immunohistochemistry for p16 is usually positive, indicating their HPV origins.

Follow-up and outcome data are scant. Adverse pathological features suggest aggressive behavior.

References

1. Thomas A, Necchi A, Muneer A, et al. Penile cancer. Nat Rev Dis Primers. 2021;7(1):11.
2. Stecca CE, Alt M, Jiang DM, et al. Recent advances in the management of penile cancer: a contemporary review of the literature. Oncol Ther. 2021;9(1):21–39.
3. Chaux A, Netto GJ, Rodríguez IM, et al. Epidemiologic profile, sexual history, pathologic features, and human papillomavirus status of 103 patients with penile carcinoma. World J Urol. 2013;31(4):861–7.
4. Chaux A, Velazquez EF, Amin A, et al. Distribution and characterization of subtypes of penile intraepithelial neoplasia and their association with invasive carcinomas: a pathological study of 139 lesions in 121 patients. Hum Pathol. 2012;43(7):1020–7.
5. Chaux A, Pfannl R, Rodríguez IM, et al. Distinctive immunohistochemical profile of penile intraepithelial lesions: a study of 74 cases. Am J Surg Pathol. 2011;35(4):553–62.
6. Chaux A, Han JS, Lee S, et al. Immunohistochemical profile of the penile urethra and differential expression of GATA3 in urothelial versus squamous cell carcinomas of the penile urethra. Hum Pathol. 2013;44(12):2760–7.
7. Steinestel J, Cronauer MV, Müller J, et al. Overexpression of p16(INK4a) in urothelial carcinoma in situ is a marker for MAPK-mediated epithelial-mesenchymal transition but is not related to human papillomavirus infection. PLoS One. 2013;8(5):e65189.

8. Velazquez EF, Cubilla AL. Lichen sclerosus in 68 patients with squamous cell carcinoma of the penis: frequent atypias and correlation with special carcinoma variants suggests a precancerous role. Am J Surg Pathol. 2003;27(11):1448–53.

9. Cañete-Portillo S, Sanchez DF, Fernández-Nestosa MJ, et al. Continuous spatial sequences of lichen Sclerosus, penile intraepithelial neoplasia, and invasive carcinomas: a study of 109 cases. Int J Surg Pathol. 2019;27(5):477–82.

10. Chaux A, Cubilla AL. Diagnostic problems in precancerous lesions and invasive carcinomas of the penis. Semin Diagn Pathol. 2012;29(2):72–82.

11. Oertell J, Caballero C, Iglesias M, et al. Differentiated precursor lesions and low-grade variants of squamous cell carcinomas are frequent findings in foreskins of patients from a region of high penile cancer incidence. Histopathology. 2011;58(6):925–33.

12. Guimarães GC, Cunha IW, Soares FA, et al. Penile squamous cell carcinoma clinicopathological features, nodal metastasis and outcome in 333 cases. J Urol. 2009;182(2):528–34. discussion 34.

13. Lam KY, Chan KW. Molecular pathology and clinicopathologic features of penile tumors: with special reference to analyses of p21 and p53 expression and unusual histologic features. Arch Pathol Lab Med. 1999;123(10):895–904.

14. Chaux A, Torres J, Pfannl R, et al. Histologic grade in penile squamous cell carcinoma: visual estimation versus digital measurement of proportions of grades, adverse prognosis with any proportion of grade 3 and correlation of a Gleason-like system with nodal metastasis. Am J Surg Pathol. 2009;33(7):1042–8.

15. Cubilla AL, Velazquez EF, Young RH. Epithelial lesions associated with invasive penile squamous cell carcinoma: a pathologic study of 288 cases. Int J Surg Pathol. 2004; 12(4):351–64.

16. Cubilla AL, Reuter V, Velazquez E, et al. Histologic classification of penile carcinoma and its relation to outcome in 61 patients with primary resection. Int J Surg Pathol. 2001; 9(2):111–20.

17. Masih AS, Stoler MH, Farrow GM, et al. Penile verrucous carcinoma: a clinicopathologic, human papillomavirus typing and flow cytometric analysis. Mod Pathol. 1992;5(1):48–55.

18. Stankiewicz E, Kudahetti SC, Prowse DM, et al. HPV infection and immunochemical detection of cell-cycle markers in verrucous carcinoma of the penis. Mod Pathol. 2009;22(9):1160–8.

19. Dai B, Ye DW, Kong YY, et al. Predicting regional lymph node metastasis in Chinese patients with penile squamous cell carcinoma: the role of histopathological classification, tumor stage and depth of invasion. J Urol. 2006;176(4 Pt 1):1431–5. discussion 5.

20. Cubilla AL, Lloveras B, Alejo M, et al. The basaloid cell is the best tissue marker for human papillomavirus in invasive penile squamous cell carcinoma: a study of 202 cases from Paraguay. Am J Surg Pathol. 2010;34(1):104–14.

21. Sanchez DF, Soares F, Alvarado-Cabrero I, et al. Comparison of pathologic and outcome features of classical vs. Mixed (Hybrid) Verrucous Carcinoma (VC) of Penis. A Study of 59 cases. Mod Pathol. 2017;30(2):255A.

22. Kato N, Onozuka T, Yasukawa K, et al. Penile hybrid verrucous-squamous carcinoma associated with a superficial inguinal lymph node metastasis. Am J Dermatopathol. 2000;22(4):339–43.

23. Clemente Ramos LM, García González R, Burgos Revilla FJ, et al. Hybrid tumor of the penis: is this denomination correct? Arch Esp Urol. 1998;51(8):821–3.

24. Chaux A, Soares F, Rodríguez I, et al. Papillary squamous cell carcinoma, not otherwise specified (NOS) of the penis: clinicopathologic features, differential diagnosis, and outcome of 35 cases. Am J Surg Pathol. 2010;34(2):223–30.

25. Gregoire L, Cubilla AL, Reuter VE, et al. Preferential association of human papillomavirus with high-grade histologic variants of penile-invasive squamous cell carcinoma. J Natl Cancer Inst. 1995;87(22):1705–9.

26. Cubilla AL, Velazquez EF, Young RH. Distinctive association of HPV with special types of penile squamous cell carcinoma and giant condyloma. A study of 211 cases. Mod Pathol. 2009;22(3):164A.

27. Barreto JE, Velazquez EF, Ayala E, et al. Carcinoma cuniculatum: a distinctive variant of penile squamous cell carcinoma: report of 7 cases. Am J Surg Pathol. 2007;31(1):71–5.

28. Lau P, Li Chang HH, Gomez JA, et al. A rare case of carcinoma cuniculatum of the penis in a 55-year-old. Can Urol Assoc J. 2010;4(5):E129–32.
29. Vinson MA, Okorji O, Gagucas R. Extensive presentation of penile carcinoma Cuniculatum a variant of squamous cell carcinoma with low malignant potential. Urol Case Rep. 2016;8:18–20.
30. Cubilla AL, Velazquez EF, Young RH. Pseudohyperplastic squamous cell carcinoma of the penis associated with lichen sclerosus. An extremely well-differentiated, nonverruciform neoplasm that preferentially affects the foreskin and is frequently misdiagnosed: a report of 10 cases of a distinctive clinicopathologic entity. Am J Surg Pathol. 2004;28(7):895–900.
31. Velazquez EF, Melamed J, Barreto JE, et al. Sarcomatoid carcinoma of the penis: a clinicopathologic study of 15 cases. Am J Surg Pathol. 2005;29(9):1152–8.
32. Fukunaga M, Yokoi K, Miyazawa Y, et al. Penile verrucous carcinoma with anaplastic transformation following radiotherapy. A case report with human papillomavirus typing and flow cytometric DNA studies. Am J Surg Pathol. 1994;18(5):501–5.
33. Urdiales Viedma M, Fernández Rodríguez A, Romero Díaz JA, et al. Squamous carcinoma of the penis with a rhabdoid phenotype. Arch Esp Urol. 2003;56(4):425–7.
34. Morinaga S, Nakamura S, Moro K, et al. Carcinosarcoma (carcinoma with sarcomatous metaplasia) of the penis. J Urol Pathol. 1995;3:369–76.
35. Antonini C, Zucconelli R, Forgiarini O, et al. Carcinosarcoma of penis. Case report and review of the literature. Adv Clin Pathol. 1997;1(4):281–5.
36. Qi XP, Lin GB, Zhu YL, et al. Pseudoangiosarcomatous squamous cell carcinoma of the penis: a case report with clinicopathological and human papilloma virus analyses. Zhonghua Nan Ke Xue. 2009;15(2):134–9.
37. Poblet E, Pascual A, Godínez JM, et al. Human papillomavirus-associated penile sarcomatoid carcinoma. J Cutan Pathol. 2008;35(6):559–65.
38. Chaux A, Reuter V, Lezcano C, et al. Comparison of morphologic features and outcome of resected recurrent and nonrecurrent squamous cell carcinoma of the penis: a study of 81 cases. Am J Surg Pathol. 2009;33(9):1299–306.
39. Cunha IW, Guimaraes GC, Soares F, et al. Pseudoglandular (adenoid, acantholytic) penile squamous cell carcinoma: a clinicopathologic and outcome study of 7 patients. Am J Surg Pathol. 2009;33(4):551–5.
40. Romero FR, de Castro MG, Garcia CR, et al. Adenosquamous carcinoma of the penis. Clinics (Sao Paulo). 2006;61(4):363–4.
41. Cubilla AL, Ayala MT, Barreto JE, et al. Surface adenosquamous carcinoma of the penis. A report of three cases. Am J Surg Pathol. 1996;20(2):156–60.
42. Jamieson NV, Bullock KN, Barker TH. Adenosquamous carcinoma of the penis associated with balanitis xerotica obliterans. Br J Urol. 1986;58(6):730–1.
43. Masera A, Ovcak Z, Volavsek M, et al. Adenosquamous carcinoma of the penis. J Urol. 1997;157(6):2261.
44. Layfield LJ, Liu K. Mucoepidermoid carcinoma arising in the glans penis. Arch Pathol Lab Med. 2000;124(1):148–51.
45. Costa MR, Sugita DM, Vilela MH, et al. Mucoepidermoid carcinoma of the penis: case report and literature review. Can Urol Assoc J. 2015;9(1-2):E27–9.
46. Yorita K, Kuroda N, Naroda T, et al. Penile warty mucoepidermoid carcinoma with features of stratified mucin-producing intra-epithelial lesion and invasive stratified mucin-producing carcinoma. Histopathology. 2018;72(5):867–73.
47. Cubilla AL, Reuter VE, Gregoire L, et al. Basaloid squamous cell carcinoma: a distinctive human papilloma virus-related penile neoplasm: a report of 20 cases. Am J Surg Pathol. 1998;22(6):755–61.
48. Epstein JI, Magi-Galluzzi C, Zhou M, et al. The penis and scrotum. In: Montgomery EA, editor. Tumors of the prostate gland, seminal vesicles, penis, and scrotum. AFIP atlas of tumor and non-tumor Pathology. 5th ed. Arlington, VA: American Registry of Pathology; 2020. p. 431–747.

49. Cubilla AL, Velazques EF, Reuter VE, et al. Warty (condylomatous) squamous cell carcinoma of the penis: a report of 11 cases and proposed classification of 'verruciform' penile tumors. Am J Surg Pathol. 2000;24(4):505–12.
50. Bezerra AL, Lopes A, Landman G, et al. Clinicopathologic features and human papillomavirus dna prevalence of warty and squamous cell carcinoma of the penis. Am J Surg Pathol. 2001;25(5):673–8.
51. Chaux A, Tamboli P, Ayala A, et al. Warty-basaloid carcinoma: clinicopathological features of a distinctive penile neoplasm. Report of 45 cases. Mod Pathol. 2010;23(6):896–904.
52. Cañete-Portillo S, Clavero O, Sanchez DF, et al. Medullary carcinoma of the penis: a distinctive HPV-related neoplasm: a report of 12 cases. Am J Surg Pathol. 2017;41(4):535–40.
53. Sanchez DF, Rodriguez IM, Piris A, et al. Clear cell carcinoma of the penis: an HPV-related variant of squamous cell carcinoma: a report of 3 cases. Am J Surg Pathol. 2016;40(7):917–22.
54. Mentrikoski MJ, Frierson HF Jr, Stelow EB, et al. Lymphoepithelioma-like carcinoma of the penis: association with human papilloma virus infection. Histopathology. 2014;64(2):312–5.

Chapter 3
IIIB: Characterization of Penile Cancers with Comprehensive Genomic Profiling

Jeffrey S. Ross, Joseph Jacob, and Gennady Bratslavsky

Introduction

Penile squamous cell carcinoma (PSCC) has increased in incidence in western societies, and is linked to increased frequencies of human papilloma virus (HPV) infection [1–3]. As reflected in a 5-year overall survival of 60%, the prognosis of PSCC has remained constant for decades [1–3], and routine prognostic assessment continues to rely mostly on clinicopathological factors such as histological grade, lymphovascular invasion, and lymph node metastasis [4]. The genetic and molecular biomarkers that have potential to identify patients with PSCC who are most likely to respond to a given therapy are only recently emerging. Surgery, chemotherapy, and radiation treatment have long served as the cornerstones of PSCC treatment [5–8]. More recently, the standard treatment for advanced PSCC has started to evolve from single chemotherapeutic agents to combination chemotherapy regimens, and finally, to targeted therapies enabling a personalized approach [8–11]. However, to date, no personalized medicine approach for the treatment of PSCC is being used in routine clinical practice. Moreover, the currently approved

J. S. Ross (✉)
Department of Urology, Upstate Medical University, Syracuse, NY, USA

Foundation Medicine, Cambridge, MA, USA
e-mail: jross@foundationmedicine.com; rossj@upstate.edu

J. Jacob · G. Bratslavsky
Department of Urology, Upstate Medical University, Syracuse, NY, USA
e-mail: jacobj@upstate.edu; bratslag@upstate.edu

© The Author(s), under exclusive license to Springer Nature Switzerland AG 2021
P. E. Spiess, A. Necchi (eds.), *Penile Carcinoma*,
https://doi.org/10.1007/978-3-030-82060-2_3

or recommended treatment regimens for advanced PSCC is very limited, and thus, the enrolling patients with PSCC in clinical trials has become an important approach for improving outcomes for this disease [12]. Today, it is widely believed that progress in the treatment of advanced PSCC will come from understanding PSCC biology and from translational research leading to novel management strategies. The utilization of next-generation sequencing techniques (NGS) to perform comprehensive genomic profiling (CGP) has led to the identification of driver mutations, both oncogenes and tumor suppressor genes associated with genomic pathway activations that occur in both HPV+ and HPV- PSCC [13–14]. In addition, CGP has enabled the identification of biomarkers associated with response and resistance to various immunotherapy options, including immune checkpoint inhibition (ICPI), vaccination therapy, and adoptive immune cell transfer [15]. In this chapter, we discuss the current knowledge of the biology of PSCC at the genomic level and evaluate new findings in the field of immuno-oncology and their potential implications for the management of clinically advanced and metastatic PSCC.

Genomic Assessment Techniques in PSCC

Genomic assessment techniques in PSCC have included limited germline genetic studies, single gene assessments, multiplex gene panels, targeted genomic profiling using next-generation sequencing methods, whole transcriptome analyses, gene expression profiles, proteomic analyses, epigenetic measurements, and microbiome evaluations [14–15]. This chapter is focused on the use of comprehensive genomic profiling, and is based on results from sequencing the extracted DNA from formalin-fixed paraffin-embedded samples from both primary tumors and metastatic sites in patients with clinically advanced PSCC (Fig. 3.1). All samples

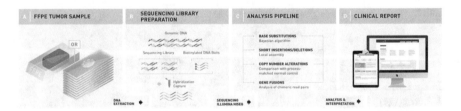

Fig. 3.1 Diagram of the hybrid capture-based DNA sequencing assay that was used to generate data is discussed in this chapter. For each PSCC case, ≥50 ng DNA was extracted from 40 μm of FFPE sections, and sequencing was performed on 324 cancer-related genes and introns from 28 genes commonly rearranged in cancer. The FDA-approved test, FoundationOne CDx used hybrid capture-based sequencing with adaptor ligation-based libraries to mean coverage depth > 600×. Tumor mutational burden (TMB) was determined on 0.8 Mb of sequenced DNA, and microsatellite instability high (MSI-high) was determined on 95 loci

forwarded for DNA extraction contained a minimum of 20% tumor cells. The samples were assayed using adaptor-ligation and hybrid capture next-generation sequencing for all coding exons from up to 324 cancer-related genes, plus select introns from up to 31 genes frequently rearranged in cancer. Patient samples were sequenced and evaluated for genomic alterations including base substitutions, insertions, deletions, copy number alterations (amplifications and homozygous deletions), and for select gene fusions/rearrangements, as previously described [16, 17]. The bioinformatics processes used in this study included Bayesian algorithms to detect base substitutions, local assembly algorithms to detect short insertions and deletions, a comparison with process-matched normal control samples to detect gene copy number alterations, and an analysis of chimeric read pairs to identify gene fusions as previously described [18]. To help visualize the sequencing data results, an oncoPrint plot was generated with the online tools of the cBioPortal as described by Gao et al. [19] and Cerami et al. [20]. Tumor mutational burden (TMB) was determined on 0.83–1.14 Mb of sequenced DNA using a mutation burden estimation algorithm that, based on the genomic alterations detected, extrapolates to the exome or the genome as a whole as previously described [21]. Assessment of microsatellite instability was performed from DNA sequencing across 114 loci, as previously described [22]. In this database, PD-L1 expression was also determined on subsets of the tumors using the DAKO 22C3 assay with low-positive tumor cell scoring defined as 1% to 49% staining and high-positive tumor cell scoring defined as ≥50% staining.

Using Comprehensive Genomic Profiling to Assist in the Management of Clinically Advanced and Metastatic PSCC

Currently Untargetable Genes

A number of studies on the genomic basis of PSCC have been published (Table 3.1) [23–32]. These studies have generally combined HPV-positive and HPV-negative cases. Currently for non-targetable genomic alterations covered in these reports, the predominant mutations have involved the *TP53* and *TERT* genes. When comprehensive genomic profiling of PSCC is divided into HPV-positive and HPV-negative cases (Fig. 3.2), these two mutations are significantly increased in the HPV-negative PSCC cases. It is believed that a significant proportion of these HPV-negative PSCC cases may have lost their HPV-positive status during disease progression as the tumor cell cycle becomes dysregulated by accumulated mutations [33–34].

Table 3.1 Studies investigating the genomic landscape of PSCC

Study year	Disease characteristics	Sample number	Analysis method	Key findings	Ref.
2001 [a]	26 patients with non-metastatic invasive PSCC (17 with lymph node invasion; 7 well-differentiated and 19 moderately differentiated primary tumours)	26 fresh-frozen samples	CGH	Most common CNA gains in 8q24, 16p11–12, 20q11–13, 22q, 19q13 and 5p15; most common deletions in 13q21–22, 4q21–32 and X chromosome	Alves et al. [31]
2007	28 patients with primary PSCC (6 pT1N0, 3 pT2N0, 3 pT3N0, 15 pTanyN1–3 M0 and 1 pTN1M1; tumour grade I in 4, II in 17 and III in 7)	38 FFPE samples (28 primary tumour, 9 lymph node metastases and 1 cutaneous metastasis)	Microsatellite-based multiplex PCR (with 62 PCR primer pairs)	LOH in >25% of primary PSCC tumours; high LOH frequency (>10) associated with occurrence of metastasis	Poetsch et al. [32]
				LOH in the region of CDKN2A (9p21) and NOL7 (6p22–23) associated with increased risk of lymph node metastases	
2015	46 patients with PSCC (clinical stage I in 12, II in 12, III in 12 and IV in 6, no data for 4 tumours); 16 patients with positive HPV genotyping (HPV16 in 12, HPV53 in 1, both HPV16 and HPV40 in 1, both HPV16 and HPV62 in 1, both HPV18 and HPV40 in 1); 7 deaths after a median of 9.7 months	46 fresh-frozen samples	Array-based CGH combined with HPV genotyping	Distinct genomic profile between HPV-positive and HPV-negative samples	Busso-Lopes et al. [33]
				Losses on 3p21.1–p14.3 and gains on 3q25.31–q29 associated with poor prognosis and survival	
				Genes on chromosome 3, such as TNFSF10 and PPARF, substantially altered and both might be novel therapeutic targets	
2016	27 patients with PSCC in the study cohort (9 HPV-positive, lymph node invasion in 12) and 70 in the validation cohort (18 HPV-positive, lymph node invasion in 30)	27 fresh-frozen samples (24 tumour–germline pairs and 3 single tumours) in the study cohort; 20 fresh-frozen and 50 FFPE samples in the validation cohort	Whole-exome sequencing	Mean somatic mutation rate per tumour, 30; non-silent mutation rates per Mb, 1.78 (range 0.72–7.5)	Feber et al. [34]
				Tumours with high HPV load had significantly reduced mutational load ($P < 0.05$)	
				HPV-associated APOBEC mutation signature significantly increased in HPV-positive samples ($P < 2.2e{-}16$)	
				GPS1 identified as a novel tumour suppressor gene and pathogenic driver	

Table 3.1 (continued)

Year	Patients	Samples	Method	Findings	Reference
2015 [b]	43 patients with PSCC (clinical stage I in 12, II in 13, III in 3 and IV in 14; tumour grade low in 13, low–moderate in 2, moderate in 19, moderate–poor in 6 and poor in 4; no primary tumour available in 1 patient with metastasis)	60 FFPE samples (14 matched primary–metastasis pairs)	Targeted, multiplexed PCR-based NGS (ion torrent Oncomine comprehensive assays; 2462 amplicons targeting 126 genes)	Most frequent CNA gains in *MYC* (11 samples), *CCND1* (8 samples), *SOX2* (8 samples), *ATP11B* (5 samples), *EGFR* (6 samples) and *TERT* (4 samples); most frequent losses in *CDKN2A* (13 samples) Amplifications in *EGFR* and *CDK4* detected, for which targeted therapies are available	McDaniel et al. [37]
2016	20 patients with advanced PSCC (tumour stage III in 3 and IV in 17; 3 HPV-positive: 2 HPV16 and 1 HPV6)	20 FFPE samples	Hybridization-captured, adaptor ligation-based, NGS (HiSeq technology Illumina; all coding exons of 236 cancer-related genes plus select introns from 19 genes)	At least one clinically relevant alteration in 19 samples (95%) Mutually exclusive *PIK3CA* and *FBXW7* alterations in 5 and 2 patients, respectively, which can be targeted with mTOR inhibitor	Ali et al. [51]
2019	78 patients with metastatic PSCC	78 FFPE samples (41 primary tumour and 37 unmatched samples from 37 metastatic sites)	Hybridization-captured, adaptor ligation-based, NGS (HiSeq technology Illumina; all coding exons from 287 to 315 cancer-related genes plus select introns from 19 to 28 genes)	Potentially targetable genomic alterations in the mTOR pathway (*NF1* in 7%, *PTEN* in 4%), in the DNA repair pathway (*BRCA2* in 7%, *ATM* in 7%) and tyrosine kinase receptors (*EGFR* in 6%, *FGFR3* in 4%, *ERBB2* in 4%) Microsatellite-high status and *CD274* (PDL1) amplification extremely rare in metastatic PSCC	Jacob et al. [40]

CNA copy number alteration, *FFPE* formalin-fixed, paraffin-embedded, *HPV* human papillomavirus, *LOH* loss of heterozygosity, *mTOR* mechanistic target of rapamycin

a First comparative genomic hybridization (CGH) study in penile squamous cell carcinoma (PSCC)

b First next-generation sequencing (NGS) study in PSCC

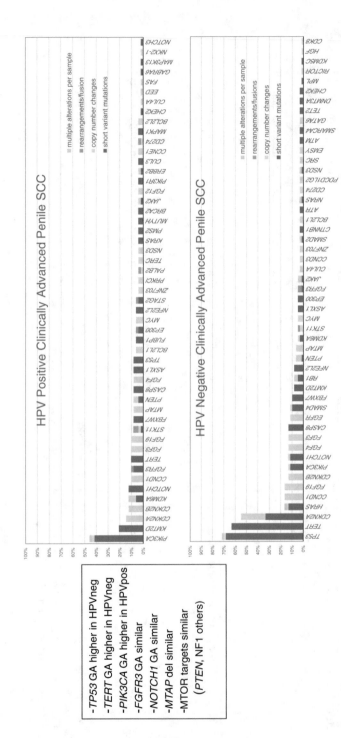

Fig. 3.2 Long tail plots of genomic alterations in HPV-positive (48 Cases) and HPV-negative (60 cases) PSCC. The frequencies of genomic alterations reveal differences between the two patient groups. The frequencies of *TP53* and *TERT* GA were higher in the HPVneg PSCC, and *PIK3CA* GA were more often identified in the in HPV-positive cases. GA in *FGFR3*, *NOTCH1*, *MTAP*, *PTEN*, and *NF1* were similar in both groups

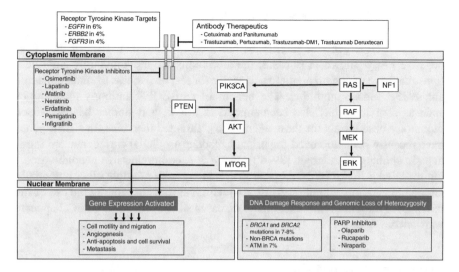

Fig. 3.3 Genomic pathways frequently activated in PSCC. GA in the MTOR, DNA repair, and tyrosine kinase receptor pathways are highlighted. (This figure is modified from Aydin et al. [14]

Targetable Genes and Pathways

The multiple genomic studies of PSCC have in common identified a variety of alterations in individual genes and genomic pathways (Fig. 3.3) that have had potential to individualize treatment for patients with clinically advanced disease [14].

MTOR Pathway

Genomic studies of PSCC have identified alterations of MTOR pathway genes such as NF1/NF2 and PTEN in 4–7% of cases [23–32]. Approved drugs such as everolimus have been approved in ongoing estrogen receptor-positive breast cancer and clinical trials using both MTOR and MEK inhibitors for MTOR pathway alterations in other tumor types [35–36].

PIK3CA

The recent approval of alpelisib for the treatment of *PIK3CA* mutated estrogen receptor-positive breast cancer has encouraged further clinical research into expanding PIK3CA inhibitors into the treatment regimens of other cancer types [37]. Activating *PIK3CA* mutations were identified in 42% on HPV-positive PSCC but only in 12% of HPV-negative PSCC (Fig. 3.2).

EGFR and *FGFR3* and Other Targetable Kinases

Although *EGFR* genomic alterations are seen in more than 10% of the HPV-negative PSCC shown in Fig. 3.2, the alterations are predominantly amplifications that have uncertain predictive capacity for responsiveness to small molecule anti-EGFR kinase inhibitors. The benefit of anti-EGFR antibody therapeutics such as cetuximab has also been limited in PSCC, and studies have not used biomarker-based trials for these agents [38]. Targeted therapies for *FGFR* genes have recently been approved for urinary bladder urothelial carcinoma and intrahepatic cholangiocarcinoma [39–40]. In *Case 1*, comprehensive genomic profiling revealed a *FGFR3-TACC3* gene fusion along with multiple other potentially targetable genomic alterations (Fig. 3.4). Clinical trials expanding the use of the new FGFR inhibitors into uncommon diseases such as metastatic PSCC appears warranted.

NOTCH Signaling Pathway

Researchers have been working on targeting tumors driven by alterations in the NOTCH family or receptors for many years. A challenge for this program has been the fact that some *NOTCH* gene mutations are activating and function like driver oncogenes and other NOTCH mutations are inactivating and function like driver tumor suppressor genes. Squamous cell carcinomas are particularly associated with *NOTCH* gene mutations [41]. In the current dataset, *NOTCH1* genomic alterations, a mix of both activating and inactivation mutations, is found in 11–12% of both HPV-positive and HPV-negative PSCC (Fig. 3.2). Recently, there appears to have been progress in the development of anti-NOTCH treatment strategies (Fig. 3.5) [41]. Interestingly, the sequencing of the tumor shown in *Case 1*, in addition to the *FGFR3* fusion alteration, also revealed both a *NOTCH1* activating mutation and a *NOTCH1-SEC16A* fusion increasing the therapy options for patients with clinically advanced metastatic PSCC (Fig. 3.4).

Homologous Recombination Defect and *BRCA*1/2 Status

Inactivating mutations in the *BRCA1* and *BRCA2* genes in PSCC are uncommon both as germline mutations and somatic tumor cell mutations [42–44]. In the current database (Fig. 3.2), *BRCA1, BRCA2,* and *ATM* mutations that have been associated with DNA damage response defects and homologous DNA repair deficiency were uniformly uncommon, although *BRCA2* mutations were identified in 4% of HPV-positive PSCC cases and *ATM* mutations were found in 3% of HPV-negative PSCC cases.

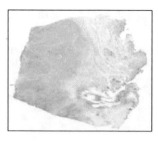
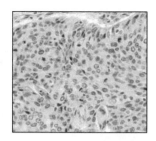
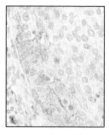

Low and high magnification of penectomy specimen with PD-L1 IHC staining (Dako 22C3)

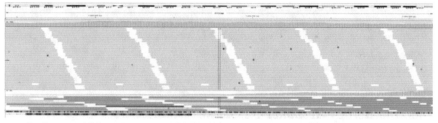

Int Genome Viewer depiction of FGFR3(NM_000142)-TACC3(NM_006342) fusion

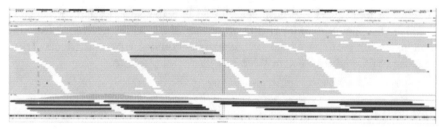

Int Genome Viewer depiction of NOTCH1(NM_017617)-SEC16A(NM_014866) fusion

Fig. 3.4 *Case 1.* Partial penectomy specimen showing high-grade SCC in a 70-year old man which progressed to metastatic disease. CGP revealed an MS stable tumor, TMB of five mutations/ Mb. There were two genomic fusions: an *FGFR3-TACC3* fusion and a *NOTCH1-SEC16A* fusion. Additional mutations were found in *NOTCH1*, *MSH6*, and *PTEN*. This tumor was P16 IHC positive, but HPV virions were not detected in the DNA sequencing procedure. PD-L1 IHC staining was focal and weak in tumor cells (1%–49%). Drugs targeting *FGFR* fusions have been approved in cholangiocarcinoma and urothelial carcinoma. Small molecule and antibody drugs targeting *NOTCH1* are in mid and late stages of clinical development

Gamma Secretase Inhibitors Phase I - Crenigestat Gamma Secretase Inhibitors Phase II - AL101 - RO4929097 Gamma Secretase Inhibitors Phase III - Nirogacestat	Monoclonal Antibodies Phase I - Enoticumumab - Brontictuzumab - MEDI0639 Monoclonal Antibodies Phase II - Demcizumab - Terextumab	Antibody Conjugates Phase I - PF-06650808 Antibody Conjugates Phase III - Rovalpituzumab teserine

Fig. 3.5 NOTCH pathway and anti-NOTCH inhibitors in early and late stages of clinical development. This figure lists the NOTCH drugs including gamma secretase inhibitors, monoclonal antibodies, and antibody conjugates in various stages of clinical development

Table 3.2 Comparison of immuno-oncology drug response associated biomarkers in HPV Pos and HPV Neg Penile SCC

	HPVposPenile SCC (48 cases)	HPVnegPenile SCC (60 cases)	P value
MSI High Status	2%	1%	NS
Mean Tumor Mutational Burden	9.0	5.6	p=.008
TMB ≥ 10 mutations/Mb	31%	12%	NS
CD274(PD-L1) Gene Amplification	4%	3%	NS
PD-L1 Low (1-49%) Expression	38%[a]	22%[b]	NS
PD-L1 High (≥50%) Expressionv	19%[a]	59%[b]	p<.0001
STK11 Short Variant Mutation	8%	5%	NS
MDM2 Amplification	<1%	<1%	NS

[a] **26 cases tested**
[b] 27 cases tested

Immunotherapy Response-Associated Biomarkers

A series of biomarkers that have been linked to responsiveness and resistance to immune checkpoint inhibitor (ICPI) treatments in PSCC are developed from the comprehensive profiling of the two separate cohorts of HPV-positive and HPV-negative PSCC and are listed in Table 3.2.

MSI Status

Microsatellite instability high status is extremely uncommon in PSCC cases ranging from 1–2% in both HPV-positive and HPV-negative cases. Hypermutated PSCC is also extremely uncommon.

TMB Status

As seen in a variety of SCC originating from other sites, the tumor mutational burden levels in PSCC are relatively high. The nine mutations per megabase of sequenced DNA mean TMB seen in the HPV-positive PSCC is significantly higher than that seen in HPV-negative cases ($p = 0.008$). Currently, a TMB of ≥10 mutations/Mb is approved by the US FDA as a pangenomic companion diagnostic for the clinical selection of pembrolizumab in solid tumors [45]. Thus, when based only on TMB levels, 31% of HPV-positive PSCC cases would be on label for ICPI-based immunotherapy, whereas only 12% of HPV-negative PSCC cases would be on label.

Genomic Alterations Associated with ICPI Responsiveness: *CD274* Amplification

In *Case 2*, a clinically advanced PSCC progressed after chemoradiation treatments. Comprehensive genomic profiling of the original primary tumors revealed an amplification of the *CD274/PD-L1* gene (Fig. 3.6). This tumor also featured 100% membranous tumor cell staining for PD-L1 expression. PD-L1 gene amplification has generally correlated with PD-L1 expression measured with immunohistochemistry [45] and has been associated as a major biomarker predictive of positive response to ICPI treatments in a wide variety of solid tumors [46].

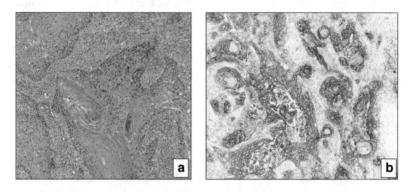

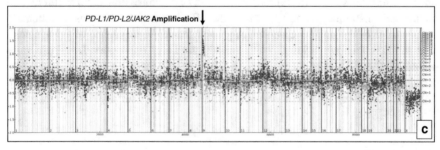

Fig. 3.6 *Case 2*. PSCC in a 73-year-old man. This clinically advanced tumor was a moderately differentiated HPV-negative keratinizing SCC with invasion into the corpora cavernosum as shown in the hematoxylin and eosin microscopic image of this penectomy specimen (**a**). The tumor cells also showed a 100% diffuse membranous pattern when stained with the Dako 22C3 anti-PD-L1 immunohistochemistry system (**b**). The tumor recurred systemically and was resistant to chemoradiation therapy. The copy number plot (**c**) shown below from the comprehensive genomic profiling performed on the primary tumor revealed amplification of multiple genes including *CD274 (PD-L1)*, *PDCD1LG2 (PD-L2)*, and *JAK2*. CD274 (PD-L1) amplification has been associated with high expression of PD-L1 detected by immunohistochemistry and increased responsiveness to immune checkpoint inhibitor-based therapy regimens

Genomic Alterations Associated with Resistance

Whereas lack of MSI-high and TMB > 10 mutations/Mb as well as absence of PD-L1 expression (see below) would be considered to be negative predictors of ICPI response, currently, there are no single gene/stand-alone biomarkers predictive of ICPI resistance approved for routine clinical use by any regulatory authority. Among potential ICPI resistance-associated genes that have been studied in tumor types other than PSCC, inactivating mutations in the *STK11* tumor suppressor gene and amplification of *MDM2* cell cycle regulatory gene are the most studied. *STK11* mutations have been linked to resistance to immunotherapy in NSCLC cases that are also positive for a *KRAS* mutation [47]. *MDM2* amplification has not been associated with resistance to ICPI in a wide variety of tumor types; *MDM2* amplification may be indicative of risk for disease hyperprogression when immunotherapy regimens are selected for treatment [48]. *STK11* mutations were found in 8% of HPV-positive PSCC (Table 3.2), but the clinical significance of this finding in this disease setting is currently unknown. *MDM2* amplification is extremely rare (<1%) in PSCC.

PD-L1 Expression

In studies of PSCC, the reported frequency of PD-L1 expression has varied from 40% and 62% [48–50]. The impact of HPV status in these studies has conflicted. In the database shown in Table 3.2, high PD-L1 expression (>50% tumor cell membranous staining using the Dako 22C3 IHC assay) at 59% was significantly greater in the HPV-negative cohort. A greater than 80% incidence of PD-L1 positive status is seen when low (1–49%) and high PD-L1 expression levels are combined in the HPV-negative group. A high concordance in PD-L1 expression between matched primary and metastatic PSCC samples has been seen [50]. Finally, PD-L1 expression has been associated with poor survival in HPV-negative PSCC [49].

Implications of Genomic Profile Differences between HPV-Positive and HPV-Negative PSCC

As seen in Fig. 3.2 and Table 3.2, there are significant differences in the genomic alterations, activated pathways and potential responses to immunotherapies based on the HPV status of PSCC. An important concept in evaluating this comparison is that when genomic evaluation of a PSCC sample reveals an HPV-negative genotype, this result may often be obtained in a later stage tumor sample which is now driven/co-driven by inactivation of the TP53 tumor suppressor gene and that the initial primary tumor early in the disease course may have actually tested as

HPV-positive. However, regardless as to how tumor cell cycle is being disrupted, HPV status appears to influence and respond to therapies including both chemotherapy [51, 52] and radiation [53].

Comparison of Genomic Alterations in PSCC with Male Urethral SCC (UrthSCC)

Although male urethral SCC may have gross and microscopic similarities with PSCC, there are significant genomic differences between these two diseases. As seen in Table 3.3, PSCC features significantly higher frequencies of HPV-positive status, *CDKN2A* deletion, *TERT* promoter inactivation, *NOTCH1* mutations, and PD-L1 high expression level than seen in UrthSCC.

Summary and Conclusions

The incidence of PSCC has increased in developed countries, likely associated with both increased HPV exposure and other environmental factors. For PSCC patients whose disease relapses or progresses after surgical resection, effective treatment options for clinically advanced and metastatic disease are limited. For the patients with advanced local and metastatic PSCC, the prognosis is dismal, and new

Table 3.3 Penile SCC vs male urethral SCC

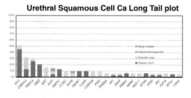

Urethral Squamous Cell Ca Long Tail plot

	Penile SCC	Male Urethral SCC	P Value
Median age (range), years	65 (24–92)	63 (40–76)	NS
GAs/tumor	5.7	4.9	NS
HPV-6/11	3%	0%	NS
HPV-16/18	29%	12%	NS
BRCA1	<1%	0%	NS
BRCA2	3%	0%	NS
CCND1 amplification	15%	6%	NS
CD274 amplification	6%	0%	NS
CDKN2A inactivation	47%	24%	P = 0.08
CDKN2B inactivation	9%	0%	NS
EGFR amplification	14%	12%	NS
FBXW7	8%	6%	NS
FGFR3	3%	6%	NS
NOTCH1	17%	0%	P = 0.08
PIK3CA	22%	30%	NS
PTEN inactivation	4%	6%	NS
TERT promoter mutation	44%	13%	P = 0.01
TP53	55%	59%	NS
MSI High	1%	0%	NS
Median TMB	3.8	3.8	NS
Mean TMB	5.7	6.5	NS
TMB ≥10 mt/Mb	15%	6%	NS
TMB >20 mt/Mb	5%	6%	NS
PD-L1 Low Positive (1-49%)	25%	28%	NS
PD-L1 High Positive (≥50%)	34%	14%	P = 0.06

management approaches are urgently needed. Recently, genomic studies have detailed the molecular landscape of PSCC. HPV-positive and HPV-negative PSCC feature both common and unique genomic alterations that can impact all types of therapies including chemotherapy, radiations therapy, targeted therapy, and immunotherapy options for the disease. When comprehensive genomic profiling is performed on PSCC samples, approximately one-third of patients with clinically advanced and metastatic disease have clinically actionable genomic alterations in a range of potential targets, including the MTOR, NOTCH signaling, DNA repair, and receptor tyrosine kinase pathways. In addition, 40–60% of PSCC tumors' varying degrees PD-L1 expression detected by immunohistochemistry which when combined with a relatively high frequency of higher tumor mutational burden indicates the strong potential of benefit for immune checkpoint inhibitor-based treatment regimens for patients with relapsed and progressive disease.

References

1. Hansen BT, Orumaa M, Lie AK, Brennhovd B, Nygård M. Trends in incidence, mortality and survival of penile squamous cell carcinoma in Norway 1956-2015. Int J Cancer. 2018;142(8):1586–93.
2. Pham MN, Deal AM, Ferguson JE 3rd, Wang Y, Smith AB, Nielsen ME et al. Contemporary survival trends in penile cancer: results from the National Cancer Database. Urol Oncol. 2017;35(12):674.e1.
3. Arya M, Li R, Pegler K, Sangar V, Kelly JD, Minhas S, Muneer A, et al. Long-term trends in incidence, survival and mortality of primary penile cancer in England. Cancer Causes Control. 2013;24(12):2169–76.
4. Ficarra V, Akduman B, Bouchot O, Palou J, Tobias-Machado M. Prognostic factors in penile cancer. Urology. 2010;76(2 Suppl 1):S66–73.
5. Veeratterapillay R, Teo L, Asterling S, Greene D. Oncologic outcomes of penile cancer treatment at a UK Supraregional center. Urology. 2015;85(5):1097–103.
6. Horenblas S. Lymphadenectomy for squamous cell carcinoma of the penis. Part 2: the role and technique of lymph node dissection. BJU Int. 2001;88(5):473–83.
7. Pagliaro LC, Williams DL, Daliani D, Williams MB, Osai W, Kincaid M, et al. Neoadjuvant paclitaxel, ifosfamide, and cisplatin chemotherapy for metastatic penile cancer: a phase II study. J Clin Oncol. 2010;28(24):3851–7.
8. Nicholson S, Hall E, Harland SJ, Chester JD, Pickering L, Barber J, et al. Phase II trial of docetaxel, cisplatin and 5FU chemotherapy in locally advanced and metastatic penis cancer (CRUK/09/001). Br J Cancer. 2013;109(10):2554–9.
9. Haas GP, Blumenstein BA, Gagliano RG, Russell CA, Rivkin SE, Culkin DJ, et al. Cisplatin, methotrexate and bleomycin for the treatment of carcinoma of the penis: a Southwest Oncology Group study. J Urol. 1999;161(6):1823–5.
10. Carthon BC, Ng CS, Pettaway CA, Pagliaro LC. Epidermal growth factor receptor-targeted therapy in locally advanced or metastatic squamous cell carcinoma of the penis. BJU Int. 2014;113(6):871–7.
11. Necchi A, Giannatempo P, Lo Vullo S, Raggi D, Nicolai N, Colecchia M, et al. Panitumumab treatment for advanced penile squamous cell carcinoma when surgery and chemotherapy have failed. Clin Genitourin Cancer. 2016;14(3):231–6.
12. Canter DJ, Nicholson S, Watkin N, Hall E, Pettaway C, InPACT Executive Committee. The International Penile Advanced Cancer Trial (InPACT): rationale and current status. Eur Urol Focus. 2019;5(5):706–9.

13. Subramaniam DS, Liu SV, Giaccone G. Novel approaches in cancer immunotherapy. Discov Med. 2016;21(116):267–74.
14. Aydin AM, Chahoud J, Adashek JJ, Azizi M, Magliocco A, Ross JS, et al. Understanding genomics and the immune environment of penile cancer to improve therapy. Nat Rev Urol. 2020;17(10):555–70.
15. Shaw KRM, Maitra A. The status and impact of clinical tumor genome sequencing. Annu Rev Genomics Hum Genet. 2019;20:413–32. https://doi.org/10.1146/annurev-genom-083118-015034. Epub 2019 Apr 17. PMID: 30995147.
16. Lipson D, Capelletti M, Yelensky R, Otto G, Parker A, Jarosz M, et al. Identification of new ALK and RET gene fusions from colorectal and lung cancer biopsies. Nat Med. 2012; 18(3):382–4.
17. He J, Abdel-Wahab O, Nahas MK, Wang K, Rampal RK, Intlekofer AM, et al. Integrated genomic DNA/RNA profiling of hematologic malignancies in the clinical setting. Blood. 2016;127(24):3004–14. https://doi.org/10.1182/blood-2015-08-664649.
18. Frampton GM, Fichtenholtz A, Otto GA, Wang K, Downing SR, He J, et al. Development and validation of a clinical cancer genomic profiling test based on massively parallel DNA sequencing. Nat Biotechnol. 2013;31(11):1023–31.
19. Gao J, Aksoy BA, Dogrusoz U, Dresdner G, Gross B, Sumer SO, et al. Integrative analysis of complex cancer genomics and clinical profiles using the cBioPortal. Sci Signal. 2013;6(269):pl1.
20. Cerami E, Gao J, Dogrusoz U, Gross BE, Sumer SO, Aksoy BA, et al. The cBio cancer genomics portal: an open platform for exploring multidimensional cancer genomics data. Cancer Discov. 2012;2(5):401–4.
21. Chalmers ZR, Connelly CF, Fabrizio D, Gay L, Ali SM, Ennis R, et al. Analysis of 100,000 human cancer genomes reveals the landscape of tumor mutational burden. Genome Med. 2017;9(1):34.
22. Trabucco SE, Gowen K, Maund SL, Sanford E, Fabrizio DA, Hall MJ, et al. A novel next-generation sequencing approach to detecting microsatellite instability and Pan-tumor characterization of 1000 microsatellite instability-high cases in 67,000 patient samples. J Mol Diagn. 2019;21(6):1053–66.
23. Alves G, Heller A, Fiedler W, Campos MM, Claussen U, Ornellas AA, et al. Genetic imbalances in 26 cases of penile squamous cell carcinoma. Genes Chromosomes Cancer. 2001;31(1):48–53.
24. Poetsch M, Schuart BJ, Schwesinger G, Kleist B, Protzel C. Screening of microsatellite markers in penile cancer reveals differences between metastatic and nonmetastatic carcinomas. Mod Pathol. 2007;20(10):1069–77.
25. Busso-Lopes AF, Marchi FA, Kuasne H, Scapulatempo-Neto C, Trindade-Filho JC, de Jesus CM, et al. Genomic profiling of human penile carcinoma predicts worse prognosis and survival. Cancer Prev Res (Phila). 2015;8(2):149–56.
26. Feber A, Worth DC, Chakravarthy A, de Winter P, Shah K, Arya M, et al. CSN1 somatic mutations in penile squamous cell carcinoma. Cancer Res. 2016;76(16):4720–7.
27. Ceulemans S, van der Ven K, Del-Favero J. Targeted screening and validation of copy number variations. Methods Mol Biol. 2012;838:311–28.
28. Li W, Olivier M. Current analysis platforms and methods for detecting copy number variation. Physiol Genomics. 2013;45(1):1–16. https://doi.org/10.1152/physiolgenomics.00082.2012.
29. McDaniel AS, Hovelson DH, Cani AK, Liu CJ, Zhai Y, Zhang Y, et al. Genomic profiling of penile squamous cell carcinoma reveals new opportunities for targeted therapy. Cancer Res. 2015;75(24):5219–27.
30. Seed G, Yuan W, Mateo J, Carreira S, Bertan C, Lambros M, et al. Gene copy number estimation from targeted next-generation sequencing of prostate cancer biopsies: analytic validation and clinical qualification. Clin Cancer Res. 2017;23(20):6070–7.
31. Hieronymus H, Murali R, Tin A, Yadav K, Abida W, Moller H, et al. Tumor copy number alteration burden is a pan-cancer prognostic factor associated with recurrence and death. elife. 2018;7:e37294.

32. Jacob JM, Ferry EK, Gay LM, Elvin JA, Vergilio JA, Ramkissoon S, et al. Comparative genomic profiling of refractory and metastatic penile and nonpenile cutaneous squamous cell carcinoma: implications for selection of systemic therapy. J Urol. 2019;201(3):541–8.

33. Mannweiler S, Sygulla S, Winter E, Regauer S. Two major pathways of penile carcinogenesis: HPV-induced penile cancers overexpress p16ink4a, HPV-negative cancers associated with dermatoses express p53, but lack p16ink4a overexpression. J Am Acad Dermatol. 2013;69(1):73–81.

34. Sharpless NE, DePinho RA. The INK4A/ARF locus and its two gene products. Curr Opin Genet Dev. 1999;9(1):22–30.

35. Chavez-MacGregor M, Gonzalez-Angulo AM. Everolimus in the treatment of hormone receptor-positive breast cancer. Expert Opin Investig Drugs. 2012;21(12):1835–43.

36. Zhou H, Luo Y, Huang S. Updates of mTOR inhibitors. Anti Cancer Agents Med Chem. 2010;10(7):571–81.

37. Armaghani AJ, Han HS. Alpelisib in the treatment of breast cancer: a short review on the emerging clinical data. Breast Cancer (Dove Med Press). 2020;12:251–8.

38. Carthon BC, Ng CS, Pettaway CA, Pagliaro LC. Epidermal growth factor receptor-targeted therapy in locally advanced or metastatic squamous cell carcinoma of the penis. BJU Int. 2014;113(6):871–7.

39. Goyal L, Kongpetch S, Crolley VE, Bridgewater J. Targeting FGFR inhibition in cholangiocarcinoma. Cancer Treat Rev. 2021;95:102170.

40. Kardoust Parizi M, Margulis V, Lotan Y, Mori K, Shariat SF. Fibroblast growth factor receptor: a systematic review and meta-analysis of prognostic value and therapeutic options in patients with urothelial bladder carcinoma. Urol Oncol. 2021;S1078–1439(21)00048-X.

41. Moore G, Annett S, McClements L, Robson T. Top Notch targeting strategies in cancer: a detailed overview of recent insights and current perspectives. Cells. 2020;9(6):1503. https://doi.org/10.3390/cells9061503. PMID: 32575680; PMCID: PMC7349363.

42. Schettini F, Giudici F, Bernocchi O, Sirico M, Corona SP, Giuliano M, et al. Poly (ADP-ribose) polymerase inhibitors in solid tumours: systematic review and meta-analysis. Eur J Cancer. 2021;149:134–52.

43. Chan CY, Tan KV, Cornelissen B. PARP inhibitors in cancer diagnosis and therapy. Clin Cancer Res. 2021;27(6):1585–94.

44. Cetin B, Wabl CA, Gumusay O. The DNA damaging revolution. Crit Rev Oncol Hematol. 2020;156:103117.

45. Huang RSP, Haberberger J, Severson E, Duncan DL, Hemmerich A, Edgerly C, et al. A pan-cancer analysis of PD-L1 immunohistochemistry and gene amplification, tumor mutation burden and microsatellite instability in 48,782 cases. Mod Pathol. 2021;34(2):252–63.

46. Goodman AM, Piccioni D, Kato S, Boichard A, Wang HY, Frampton G, et al. Prevalence of PDL1 amplification and preliminary response to immune checkpoint blockade in solid tumors. JAMA Oncol. 2018;4(9):1237–44.

47. Kato S, Goodman A, Walavalkar V, Barkauskas DA, Sharabi A, Kurzrock R. Hyperprogressors after immunotherapy: analysis of genomic alterations associated with accelerated growth rate. Clin Cancer Res. 2017;23(15):4242–50. https://doi.org/10.1158/1078-0432.CCR-16-3133.

48. Attalla K, Sfakianos JP, Galsky MD. Current role of checkpoint inhibitors in urologic cancers. Cancer Treat Res. 2018;175:241–58.

49. Ottenhof SR, Djajadiningrat RS, de Jong J, Thygesen HH, Horenblas S, Jordanova ES. Expression of programmed death ligand 1 in penile cancer is of prognostic value and associated with HPV status. J Urol. 2017;197(3 Pt 1):690–7.

50. Udager AM, Liu TY, Skala SL, Magers MJ, McDaniel AS, Spratt DE, et al. Frequent PD-L1 expression in primary and metastatic penile squamous cell carcinoma: potential opportunities for immunotherapeutic approaches. Ann Oncol. 2016;27(9):1706–12.

51. Spiess PE, Dhillon J, Baumgarten AS, Johnstone PA, Giuliano AR. Pathophysiological basis of human papillomavirus in penile cancer: key to prevention and delivery of more effective therapies. CA Cancer J Clin. 2016;66(6):481–95.

52. Stecca CE, Alt M, Jiang DM, Chung P, Crook JM, Kulkarni GS, Sridhar SS. Recent advances in the management of penile cancer: a contemporary review of the literature. Oncol Ther. 2021;9(1):21–39.
53. Bandini M, Ross JS, Zhu Y, Ye DW, Ornellas AA, Watkin N, et al. Association between human papillomavirus infection and outcome of perioperative nodal radiotherapy for penile carcinoma. Eur Urol Oncol. 2020:S2588–9311(20)30176–0.

Chapter 4
Functional and Psychosocial Impact of Penile Cancer Treatments

Grant R. Pollock, Jiping Zeng, and Juan Chipollini

Introduction

Penile cancer is a rare disease in Europe and North America, with incidence approaching 1 per 100,000 men [1]. Social and cultural habits influence the incidence of disease, which is related to exposure to the human papilloma virus (HPV) types 16 and 18, socio-economic factors, chronic irritation, phimosis, and smoking [2, 3]. Treatment goals include complete eradication of disease while preserving as much of the penis as possible [4]. Treatments for early stage disease include organ-preservation strategies, while the gold standard of therapy in patients with invasive disease is radical surgery [4, 5].

Although amputation can be curative, it can have devastating consequences for patients' mental well-being [6]. The diagnosis of penile cancer, along with the more disfiguring treatments that accompany it, can have a significant impact on the patient's quality of life, sexual function, self-image, and self-esteem [2, 7]. In this chapter, we discuss the current evidence on the psychological burden of penile cancer and the treatments that accompany it, in terms of sexual function, quality of life, and psychosocial well-being.

G. R. Pollock · J. Zeng · J. Chipollini (✉)
Department of Urology, The University of Arizona, Tucson, AZ, USA
e-mail: grantpollock@arizona.edu; jzeng1@arizona.edu; jchipollini@surgery.arizona.edu

© The Author(s), under exclusive license to Springer Nature Switzerland AG 2021   47
P. E. Spiess, A. Necchi (eds.), *Penile Carcinoma*,
https://doi.org/10.1007/978-3-030-82060-2_4

Stressors of Local Treatment

The standard treatment of penile cancer for decades has been partial and radical penectomy, both having significant consequences for patient self-esteem and body image. Recently, organ-sparing approaches for the management of low-stage penile tumors have become widely accepted due to their established oncologic control while achieving satisfactory somatic and sexual health outcomes [8–11].

A range of treatments are available for localized, early stage disease, including topical 5-Flurouracil therapy, laser therapy, glans resurfacing and glansectomy with reconstruction [2]. Surgical treatment with partial or total penectomy with or without radiotherapy is considered the gold standard for high-grade and high-stage disease [2, 4]. Additionally, patients with inguinal node disease undergo regional lymphadenectomy, which can be debilitating with complications such as lymphoedema, infection, and wound dehiscence occurring in up to 40% of individuals [2]. The rarity of the disease makes it difficult to perform prospective studies; thus, the literature is scarce in terms of comparing oncologic efficacy and functional outcomes after local treatment. Here, we summarize the relevant literature on the psychosocial and quality of life impact of penile cancer diagnosis and treatment on penile cancer patients.

Total and Partial Penectomy

Radical surgery with total or partial penectomy is the preferred method of treatment and is considered the gold standard in patients with large, high-grade and invasive tumors [4, 5]. The radical treatment of a patient's reproductive organs can add significant psychosocial burden. Additionally, the nature of radical surgery will inherently lead to a significant change in a patient's sexual health and function. Multiple studies have been performed in recent years, which document the affect that radical treatment has on both quality of life and sexual health [7].

Sexual function following partial penectomy has been reported in a few small studies [7]. With regard to penile length, one study of 18 partial penectomy patients reported a median penile flaccid length of 4 cm postoperatively [12]. Additionally, *Romero* et al. identified 55.6% of patients in their post-penectomy study as having reported erectile function suitable for intercourse posttreatment using the International Index of Erectile Function (IIEF-15) survey [12]. In patients who reported no postoperative sexual activity, 50% stated the main reason was a feeling of shame owing to the small penis size and absence of the glans [7, 12]. Two thirds of patients in this study who reported resuming sexual activity following surgery also reported a decrease in frequency of intercourse compared to preoperative frequency [12]. This study also demonstrated a decrease in sexual function following partial penectomy, with 12/18 (66.6%) patients having reduced overall satisfaction postoperatively [12].

A similar study of 14 partial penectomy patients identified 5 patients (36%) having decreased or no sexual function after partial penectomy. In this cohort, no significant levels of anxiety or depression were reported [13]. These findings were measured using the General Health Questionnaire-12 (GHQ-12) and Hospital Anxiety and Depression Scale (HADS). Social activity remained the same postoperatively; however, the authors did find the greatest difficulty men faced in the first 3 months after surgery involved difficulties with sexual activity and the discomfort with sitting to urinate. Most men reported significant stress over the fears of both mutilation and death, and the most common response to what helped them overcome these issues was the emotional support of their families [13].

Another small series of 17 patients by *Ficarra* et al. included patients treated with both partial penectomy ($n = 11$) and total penectomy ($n = 2$), as well as two patients who were nonsurgically treated with radiotherapy [14]. The authors found that patients with more mutilating treatments reported worse function. Approximately 35% of the patients reported limitations in their state of health in addition to social problems. Anxiety was prevalent following partial penectomy, as approximately 31% of patients were found to have elevated levels of anxiety postoperatively. Depression was found to be present postoperatively in 6% of patients, which was comparable to other urologic malignancies, including renal and prostate cancer [14]. Postoperative anxiety levels, however, were found to be more than double that of patients with bladder cancer who had been treated with cystectomy [14]. The authors concluded that patients undergoing partial penectomy for squamous penile carcinoma showed significant impairment in their general state of health, with anxiety being the most significant, compared with controls being treated for benign or other malignant diseases [7, 14].

Regarding reconstruction, distal reconstruction following a partial penectomy has been reported in a small series of 14 patients [15]. All patients in this study noticed thermal and tactile sensibility in the area of the neoglans, and 71% of patients noticed spontaneous and/or induced rigid erections [15]. Additionally, survey scores in the ejaculation and orgasm domains did not change postoperatively compared to preoperative functions, and no local disease recurrence or retraction was seen at 1-year postoperatively [7, 15]. Alei et al. reported ten patients who underwent partial penectomy and reconstruction with ventral fenestrated flap technique [16]. The average aesthetic satisfaction 1 month postoperatively was of 2 points, 40 months postoperatively it was of 3 points (scoring scale: 1 = complete dissatisfaction, 5 = complete satisfaction). The average IIEF score in the preoperative period was 21.6 points, 1 month postoperatively it was 13 points, 40 months postoperatively it was 19.7 points (mild erectile dysfunction) [10] (Table 4.1).

Data regarding total penile reconstruction is scarce; although it is not possible to restore full penile function, cosmetically acceptable outcomes have been noted [17–19]. *Garaffa* et al. reported a series of 15 patients who underwent total phallic reconstruction with the use of a radial artery free flap and found cosmetically acceptable results in all patients. Additionally, at a median follow-up of 20 months, all patients were satisfied with cosmesis and size of the phallus, and 14 were able to void while standing. A total of seven patients underwent inflatable penile prosthesis placement and five of these patients were subsequently able to engage in intercourse [17]. Despite these promising results, future studies on the long-term durability of total penile reconstruction are needed.

Table 4.1 Relevant studies on the psychosocial impact of radical and partial penectomy

Study	N	Treatment	Results
D'Ancona et al., *Urology* 1997 [13]	14	Partial penectomy	In 64% the overall sexual function was normal or slightly decreased; sexual interest and satisfaction remained normal or slightly reduced in 9 and 12 patients, respectively
Ficarra et al., *Prog Urol* 1999 [14]	17	Partial penectomy [11], total penectomy [4], radiotherapy [2]	The global sexual function was compromised in 76.5%; 29.5% presented with anxiety and 6% with depression
Romero et al., *Urology* 2005 [12]	18	Partial penectomy	55.6% reported erectile function that allowed sexual intercourse; 33.3% maintained their preoperative sexual intercourse frequency and were satisfied with their sexual relationship and their overall sex life
Gulino et al., *J Urol* 2007 [15]	14	Partial penectomy	71% had spontaneous and/or induced erections; IIEF scores in the ejaculation and orgasm domains did not significantly change
Alei et al., *Ann Ital Chir* 2012 [16]	10	Partial penectomy	The average IIEF score in the preoperative period was 21.6 points, 1 month postoperatively it was 13 points, 40 months postoperatively it was 19.7 points (mild erectile dysfunction)

Organ-Sparing Procedures

Conventional treatment of penile cancer has historically consisted of radical or partial penectomy with a tumor-free margin of 2 cm generally advocated [10]. Given the significant sexual and psychosocial outcomes of penile cancer treatment, there has been more widespread acceptance and utilization of penile-conserving strategies [4, 20]. From a urinary standpoint, patients undergoing radical surgery are able to void upright, but spraying does remain a common problem [21]. In one study, patients who underwent organ-sparing procedures were less likely to leak during urination compared to those undergoing partial/total penectomy (43% vs 83%), with the two most common reasons cited for the leakage being too short of a penis and spraying urine [22].

Different organ-preserving treatments are possible for noninvasive disease, including topical chemotherapy, laser therapy, Mohs micrographic surgery, external radiotherapy, brachytherapy, glans resurfacing, and glansectomy [7]. Topical 5-fluorouracil (5-FU) is a thymidylate synthase inhibitor that disrupts DNA replication, thereby exerting a cytotoxic effect on cancer cells [23]. It is regarded as a potential first-line therapy for carcinoma in situ; however, due to the rarity of this disease, there are few randomized trials to provide level 1 evidence. Local side effects appear tolerable, and include hypersensitivity and pain [23]. Systemic absorption is theoretically possible but has yet to be reported [23–25].

Laser therapy with a carbon dioxide or neodymium:YAG laser has been shown to control local disease and equivalent to other conventional organ-sparing therapies but with superior cosmetic and functional results and without compromising cure

[26, 27]. Sexual and quality of life outcomes are promising in patients treated with laser therapy. In one series of patients who underwent laser treatment for penile carcinoma, 30/40 (75%) patients who were sexually active prior to treatment reported to have resumed activity after treatment [28]. Of the entire cohort analyzed, 50% of patients reported that they were satisfied with their sexual lives following laser treatment, with only 3% of patients reporting posttreatment dyspareunia [28].

Another retrospective review found that 69% of patients showed marked decrease in some sexual practices, such as manual or oral stimulation, but a general satisfaction rate with life overall, including sexual function [8]. Another series from *van Bezooinjen* et al. found that no sexual dysfunction occurred in 19 patients who underwent laser treatment [26]. Lastly, a large study on carbon dioxide laser treatment in 224 patients showed zero reported complaints with regard to erection capability or functional impairment with sexual activity [29]. The literature shows that laser treatment is safe and effective with only marginal effects on sexual function and outcomes. There is, however, a small risk of dyspareunia and decreased libido [8, 26, 29] (Table 4.2).

There are few studies reporting sexual function and quality of life outcomes following glansectomy. Two studies have reported positive sexual outcomes following glansectomy. In one study, 79% of patients did not report any decline in spontaneous erection, rigidity, and penetrative capacity after surgery, while 75% reported recovery of orgasms [7, 30]. In another study of 12 patients, all reported a return to "normal" sexual activity 1 month after surgery [31].

Table 4.2 Relevant studies on the psychosocial impact of organ-sparing treatment

Study	N	Treatment	Results
Windahl et al., *J Urol* 2004 [28]	36	Laser	75% had resumed sexual activity; 72% reported unaltered erectile function; 50% were satisfied with their sexual life; 10% had dyspareunia; 78% considered satisfying cosmetic results
Skeppner et al., *Eur Urol* 2008 [8]	46	Laser	65% had resumed sexual activity; 75% were satisfied with life as a whole; 54% were satisfied with their sexual life; 76% were satisfied with their sexual health
Hadway et al., *BJU Int* 2006 [40]	7	Total glans resurfacing	All patients who were previously sexually active were sexually active within 3–5 months of surgery
Li et al., *Urology* 2011 [31]	29	Radical circumcision and/or wide local excision	In the group of patients with no to mild erectile dysfunction prior to surgery, 21/22 had the same rating of sexual function as before
Opjordsmoen et al., *Br J Urol* 1994 [41]	30	Local excision/laser beam treatment [5], radiotherapy [12], partial penectomy [9], total penectomy [4]	Patients treated with partial or total penectomy had a worse outcome with regard to sexual function than patients treated conservatively; 50% had mental symptoms at follow-up

Mohs micrographic surgery is another surgical option for patients with low-grade penile lesions. This method affords maximal sparing of normal penile tissue and detects tumor outgrowths, which aims at removal of the lesion with negative margins; although to date, its use is mostly for small and carcinoma in situ lesions [21]. Mohs surgery produces the most cosmetically and functionally favorable outcomes, but the rate of long-term recurrence is high [32]. Complications of Mohs surgery include meatal or urethral stenosis, as well as disfigurement of the glans [21, 33, 34]. Studies on functional outcomes for these maximal preserving strategies continue to be lacking.

Nonsurgical Strategies

From a cancer control standpoint, results of brachytherapy when compared to penectomy as primary treatment of penile cancer have been mixed [35–37]. A study by *Sarin* et al. found that brachytherapy was associated with worse oncologic outcomes when compared to penectomy, while another study by *Crook* et al. demonstrated that brachytherapy successfully treated early stage disease with survival rates similar to penectomy [36, 37]. Although there are no studies that directly observe quality of life outcomes following brachytherapy to our knowledge, well-known complications of brachytherapy include urethral stenosis and glans necrosis [35–37].

Other treatment approaches, such as external beam radiotherapy, is an available tool for smaller lesions. Radiotherapy has historically been related to complications such as chronic edema and meatal stenosis leading to decreased sexual function [38, 39]. Glans resurfacing has been described as an alternative to laser therapy in patients with noninvasive disease [7]. One study with 10 patients found that none experienced any posttreatment erectile dysfunction, and all of the patients were sexually active again within 3 to 5 months [40]. Additionally, all of the patients in the study reported that sensation at the tip of their penis was either no different or better after surgery and were able to have erections within 2–3 weeks of surgery. Overall patient satisfaction was high, and no change in penile length was documented [40].

Long-Term Outcomes

A study by *Opjordsmoen* et al. followed penile cancer patients posttreatment for a median of 80 months, and included a total of 30 patients [41]. This study observed patients who underwent local excision/laser beam treatment ($n = 5$), radiotherapy ($n = 12$), partial penectomy ($n = 9$), and total penectomy ($n = 4$). The authors found that those treated with partial or total penectomy had a worse outcome with regard to sexual function than patients treated conservatively, but there was no difference in the other domains of quality of life, indicating that even the more radically treated patients were able to adapt adequately [7, 41]. Approximately half of the patients in the cohort reported some mental symptoms at follow-up. Ultimately, 7/30 men reported that if given the opportunity to choose again, they would elect for a treatment with a lower long-term survival in order to have increased chance of remaining sexually potent [41]. The results of this study indicate that at least some penile cancer patients would prioritize short-term sexual health over long-term cancer control.

Conclusion

Penile cancer carries significant psychological impact on both patients and families. This chapter provides evidence on the effect of diagnosis and treatment of penile cancer on the psychological burden of patients and families, which is often unrecognized. Further research is required to clarify the impact of genitourinary malignancies on partners and families. Additionally, more work is required to define appropriate strategies to reduce the chance of psychological morbidity and facilitate appropriate interventions when required.

References

1. Bray F, Klint A, Gislum M, Hakulinen T, Engholm G, Tryggvadottir L, et al. Trends in survival of patients diagnosed with male genital cancers in the Nordic countries 1964-2003 followed up until the end of 2006. Acta Oncol. 2010;49(5):644–54.
2. Maddineni SB, Lau MM, Sangar VK. Identifying the needs of penile cancer sufferers: a systematic review of the quality of life, psychosexual and psychosocial literature in penile cancer. BMC Urol. 2009;9:8.
3. Dillner J, von Krogh G, Horenblas S, Meijer CJ. Etiology of squamous cell carcinoma of the penis. Scand J Urol Nephrol Suppl. 2000;205:189–93.
4. Hakenberg OW, Comperat EM, Minhas S, Necchi A, Protzel C, Watkin N, et al. EAU guidelines on penile cancer: 2014 update. Eur Urol. 2015;67(1):142–50.
5. National Comprehensive Cancer Network. NCCN Clinical Practice GUidelines in Oncology – Penile Cancer (Version 2.2017). 2017. Available online: https://www.nccn.org/professionals/physician_gls/pdf/penile.pdf.
6. Diorio GJ, Leone AR, Spiess PE. Management of Penile Cancer. Urology. 2016;96:15–21.
7. Audenet F, Sfakianos JP. Psychosocial impact of penile carcinoma. Transl Androl Urol. 2017;6(5):874–8.
8. Skeppner E, Windahl T, Andersson SO, Fugl-Meyer KS. Treatment-seeking, aspects of sexual activity and life satisfaction in men with laser-treated penile carcinoma. Eur Urol. 2008;54(3):631–9.
9. Skeppner E, Fugl-Meyer K. Dyadic aspects of sexual well-being in men with laser-treated penile carcinoma. Sex Med. 2015;3(2):67–75.
10. Lont AP, Gallee MP, Meinhardt W, van Tinteren H, Horenblas S. Penis conserving treatment for T1 and T2 penile carcinoma: clinical implications of a local recurrence. J Urol. 2006;176(2):575–80. discussion 80.

11. Djajadiningrat RS, van Werkhoven E, Meinhardt W, van Rhijn BW, Bex A, van der Poel HG, et al. Penile sparing surgery for penile cancer-does it affect survival? J Urol. 2014;192(1):120–5.
12. Romero FR, Romero KR, Mattos MA, Garcia CR, Fernandes RC, Perez MD. Sexual function after partial penectomy for penile cancer. Urology. 2005;66(6):1292–5.
13. D'Ancona CA, Botega NJ, De Moraes C, Lavoura NS, Santos JK, Rodrigues NN. Quality of life after partial penectomy for penile carcinoma. Urology. 1997;50(4):593–6.
14. Ficarra V, Mofferdin A, D'Amico A, Zanon G, Schiavone D, Malossini G, et al. Comparison of the quality of life of patients treated by surgery or radiotherapy in epidermoid cancer of the penis. Prog Urol. 1999;9(4):715–20.
15. Gulino G, Sasso F, Falabella R, Bassi PF. Distal urethral reconstruction of the glans for penile carcinoma: results of a novel technique at 1-year of followup. J Urol. 2007;178(3 Pt 1):941–4.
16. Alei G, Letizia P, Sorvillo V, Alei L, Ricottilli F, Scuderi N. Lichen sclerosus in patients with squamous cell carcinoma. Our experience with partial penectomy and reconstruction with ventral fenestrated flap. Ann Ital Chir. 2012;83(4):363–7.
17. Garaffa G, Raheem AA, Christopher NA, Ralph DJ. Total phallic reconstruction after penile amputation for carcinoma. BJU Int. 2009;104(6):852–6.
18. Gerullis H, Georgas E, Bagner JW, Eimer C, Otto T. Construction of a penoid after penectomy using a transpositioned testicle. Urol Int. 2013;90(2):240–2.
19. Hage JJ. Simple, safe, and satisfactory secondary penile enhancement after near-total oncologic amputation. Ann Plast Surg. 2009;62(6):685–9.
20. Minhas S, Kayes O, Hegarty P, Kumar P, Freeman A, Ralph D. What surgical resection margins are required to achieve oncological control in men with primary penile cancer? BJU Int. 2005;96(7):1040–3.
21. Kamel MH, Bissada N, Warford R, Farias J, Davis R. Organ sparing surgery for penile cancer: a systematic review. J Urol. 2017;198(4):770–9.
22. Kieffer JM, Djajadiningrat RS, van Muilekom EA, Graafland NM, Horenblas S, Aaronson NK. Quality of life for patients treated for penile cancer. J Urol. 2014;192(4):1105–10.
23. Longley DB, Harkin DP, Johnston PG. 5-fluorouracil: mechanisms of action and clinical strategies. Nat Rev Cancer. 2003;3(5):330–8.
24. Goette DK, Carson TE. Erythroplasia of Queyrat: treatment with topical 5-fluorouracil. Cancer. 1976;38(4):1498–502.
25. Alnajjar HM, Lam W, Bolgeri M, Rees RW, Perry MJ, Watkin NA. Treatment of carcinoma in situ of the glans penis with topical chemotherapy agents. Eur Urol. 2012;62(5):923–8.
26. van Bezooijen BP, Horenblas S, Meinhardt W, Newling DW. Laser therapy for carcinoma in situ of the penis. J Urol. 2001;166(5):1670–1.
27. Windahl T, Hellsten S. Laser treatment of localized squamous cell carcinoma of the penis. J Urol. 1995;154(3):1020–3.
28. Windahl T, Skeppner E, Andersson SO, Fugl-Meyer KS. Sexual function and satisfaction in men after laser treatment for penile carcinoma. J Urol. 2004;172(2):648–51.
29. Bandieramonte G, Colecchia M, Mariani L, Lo Vullo S, Pizzocaro G, Piva L, et al. Peniscopically controlled CO2 laser excision for conservative treatment of in situ and T1 penile carcinoma: report on 224 patients. Eur Urol. 2008;54(4):875–82.
30. Austoni EGA, Colombo F, et al. Reconstructive surgery for penile cancer with preservation of sexual function (abstract 183). Eur Urol. 2008;7:116.
31. Li J, Zhu Y, Zhang SL, Wang CF, Yao XD, Dai B, et al. Organ-sparing surgery for penile cancer: complications and outcomes. Urology. 2011;78(5):1121–4.
32. Chipollini J, Yan S, Ottenhof SR, Zhu Y, Draeger D, Baumgarten AS, et al. Surgical management of penile carcinoma in situ: results from an international collaborative study and review of the literature. BJU Int. 2018;121(3):393–8.
33. Shindel AW, Mann MW, Lev RY, Sengelmann R, Petersen J, Hruza GJ, et al. Mohs micrographic surgery for penile cancer: management and long-term followup. J Urol. 2007;178(5):1980–5.

34. Mohs FE, Snow SN, Larson PO. Mohs micrographic surgery for penile tumors. Urol Clin North Am. 1992;19(2):291–304.
35. Hasan S, Francis A, Hagenauer A, Hirsh A, Kaminsky D, Traughber B, et al. The role of brachytherapy in organ preservation for penile cancer: a meta-analysis and review of the literature. Brachytherapy. 2015;14(4):517–24.
36. Sarin R, Norman AR, Steel GG, Horwich A. Treatment results and prognostic factors in 101 men treated for squamous carcinoma of the penis. Int J Radiat Oncol Biol Phys. 1997;38(4):713–22.
37. Crook JM, Jezioranski J, Grimard L, Esche B, Pond G. Penile brachytherapy: results for 49 patients. Int J Radiat Oncol Biol Phys. 2005;62(2):460–7.
38. Edsmyr F, Andersson L, Esposti PL. Combined bleomycin and radiation therapy in carcinoma of the penis. Cancer. 1985;56(6):1257–63.
39. Gerbaulet A, Lambin P. Radiation therapy of cancer of the penis. Indications, advantages, and pitfalls. Urol Clin North Am. 1992;19(2):325–32.
40. Hadway P, Corbishley CM, Watkin NA. Total glans resurfacing for premalignant lesions of the penis: initial outcome data. BJU Int. 2006;98(3):532–6.
41. Opjordsmoen S, Fosså SD. Quality of life in patients treated for penile cancer. A follow-up study. Br J Urol. 1994;74(5):652–7.

Part II
Management of Primary Penile Tumors

Chapter 5
Penile-Sparing Surgical and Non-Surgical Approaches

Marta Skrodzka, Benjamin Ayres, and Nicholas Watkin

Abbreviations

CO_2	Carbon dioxide
HPV	Human papillomavirus
IQ	Imiquimod
KTP	Potassium titanyl phosphate
MMC	Mohs micrographic surgery
Nd:YAG	Neodymium-doped yttrium aluminium garnet
PeIN	Penile intraepithelial neoplasia
SCC	Squamous cell cancer
STSG	Split thickness skin graft
OSS	Organ-sparing surgery
TNM	Tumour nodes metastases – tumour staging classification
UICC	Union for International Cancer Control
WLE	Wide local excision

Introduction

The overall incidence of penile cancer is around 1/100000 males [1]. Significant variation is observed worldwide depending on ethnic and cultural differences, religious practices, socioeconomic status and HPV epidemiology [1, 2]. Nevertheless,

M. Skrodzka (✉) · B. Ayres · N. Watkin
St. George's University Hospital, London, UK
e-mail: marta.skrodzka@nhs.net; benjamin.ayres@nhs.net; nick.watkin@nhs.net

© The Author(s), under exclusive license to Springer Nature Switzerland AG 2021   59
P. E. Spiess, A. Necchi (eds.), *Penile Carcinoma*,
https://doi.org/10.1007/978-3-030-82060-2_5

penile cancer is a rare malignancy in developed countries [1, 2]. Due to rarity of the disease, the concept of centralised networks providing multidisciplinary approach, expertise and possibilities including research is strongly supported. Tertiary centre care is crucial to develop standardised protocols, provide optimal treatment and is proven to improve survival [3].

Historically, aggressive treatment of penile cancer resulted in penile loss and carried significant psychological burden to a penile cancer survivor. Debilitating effects of penectomy are caused by the inability to pass urine in the standing position, compromise to sexual life and an impaired sense of masculinity. High-volume centres have provided opportunities to introduce penile-preserving techniques with minimal loss of urinary and sexual function, aesthetical and psychological advancement without compromise to oncological control [4, 5].

The last 20 years has brought significant improvement in understanding of the disease changing management from aggressive, radical, mutilating surgeries to the current choice of penile-preserving, minimally invasive surgical and non-surgical options.

Non-surgical therapeutic options like topical therapy and radiotherapy were developed for low-risk, mostly superficial tumours with the aim of preserving the aesthetics and function of the organ. There was a paradigm shift in surgical options in that primarily advised surgical margin over 2 cm was proven outdated with the results of modern studies. Several publications advocated less radical surgical treatment, proving good oncological outcomes and subsequently minimising surgical margins from 10–15 mm [6], below 10 mm [7, 8], below 5 mm [9, 10] to above 1 mm [11]. These studies also identified higher tumour stage, grade, lymphovascular invasion, perineural invasion, penile intraepithelial neoplasia and positive definitive margins as risk factors for local recurrence [9, 11, 12]. What is important, however, is that in general, local recurrence can be managed surgically without negative influence on long-term survival [13, 14], although one recent study suggested that local recurrence could compromise prognosis [12]. In order to achieve optimal oncological outcomes of penile-preserving treatment, careful selection of patients, strict follow-up and patient's compliance are crucial.

When pushing the limits of penile-sparing surgery, it is also important to balance the realistic possibilities vs. patient's expectations. It is better to offer a functioning perineal urethrostomy than a short penile stump insufficient to direct urine stream and for sexual intercourse.

Penile-sparing techniques can offer expected results when tailored to individual patients. Provided that around 80% of penile cancers occur distally involving preputic and/or glans, penile-preserving surgery is feasible for large proportion of our patients [15, 16].

The degree of penile preservation depends on the time of presentation – the earlier the patient seeks doctor's advice the more likely less radical treatment is needed, and more options are possible. Delayed presentation due to fear, lack of awareness, embarrassment, and denial limits reconstructive possibilities, pushes options towards amputative surgical approaches. This is why promotion of awareness is of utmost importance and may influence final prognosis of these patients.

Penile-Sparing Conservative Therapies

Table 5.1 presents available penile-sparing approaches divided according to penile cancer staging.

Topical Chemotherapy and Immunotherapy

Indication: PeIN.

5-Fluorouracil (5-FU)

Topical chemotherapy is an effective first-line therapy in focal lesions. There is no standard protocol for the optimum treatment regimen. In our centre, we recommend 5-FU cream application for 12 hours every second day for 28 days with the advice to avoid scrotal skin involvement. Most patients will develop a degree of inflammation and/or erosion, which can be particularly unpleasant on scrotal skin [17–19]. This inflammatory process is inevitable and may reduce compliance. Topical steroids may help to alleviate the process in severe cases, but in most patients, they are not necessary. Patients need to be informed appropriately and explained that it may take several weeks for the penile mucosa to settle. Response to treatment is

Table 5.1 Penile cancer staging (eighth Edition of the UICC TNM clinical and pathological classification of penile cancer [48]) and options of penile-preserving techniques

Penile cancer stage – tumour characteristic	Penile-sparing approach
PeIN	Topical chemotherapy Topical immunotherapy Moh's micrographic surgery Laser excision/ablation Circumcision/wide local excision Glans resurfacing
pTa; pT1a (G1,G2)	Moh's micrographic surgery Laser excision/ablation Circumcision/wide local excision Glans resurfacing Glansectomy, partial glansectomy Radiotherapy in tumours <4 cm
pT1b (G3)	Glansectomy, partial glansectomy Circumcision/wide local excision Radiotherapy in tumours <4 cm
pT2	Glansectomy, partial glansectomy Wide local excision + circumcision Radiotherapy in tumours <4 cm

evaluated after this time. On rare occasions, allergic reactions may occur leading to severe dermatitis, anogenital eczema and infection [20]. This treatment should be avoided in immunocompromised patients and widespread disease [19].

Imiquimod (IQ)

In our practice, we recommend IQ immunotherapy in cases resistant, or partially responsive, to 5-FU. Some authors suggest IQ for treatment of HPV-related disease [20]. Similarly, to 5-FU, the treatment regimen is not unified, but most commonly application for 3–5 days per week for 4–6 weeks is advised.

Side effects are similar to topical chemotherapy. Rarely treatment may be complicated with systemic toxicity and hypopigmentation [18–20]. Scrotal ulceration and bleeding can be observed, and patients should be advised to avoid exposure of scrotal area to IQ [17]. Unfortunately, no large-scale long-term efficacy on IQ data is available.

The largest study of topical therapies for PeIN (5-FU and IQ as a second line) reported complete response in 57% of the patients and partial response in 13.6% at a mean follow-up of 34 months [17]. Similar outcomes were reported by other authors – of complete response in 65% and partial response in 25% at median 18 months follow-up [18]. Circumcision is a supportive measure advised in this group of patients improving response rate [17, 20]. Pre-treatment biopsy is important as 8,7% of the patients with clinical suspicion of PeIN were diagnosed with invasive SCC on biopsy or circumcision [20]. Incomplete response carries a risk of undiagnosed invasive malignancy and warrants re-biopsy or excision. Long-term surveillance is advised as minimal proportion of patients (2,6%) progress to invasive SCC [20].

Radiotherapy

Indication: Ta–T3 in tumours <4 cm.

Radiotherapy is a well-established organ-preserving technique. Modalities include external radiotherapy and brachytherapy boost or brachytherapy. Radiotherapy, especially the external beam technique, has higher recurrence rates in comparison to surgical treatment. The reported local recurrence rates are 38–43% for external beam and 13–20% for brachytherapy with the best results in pT1-pT2 tumours [21, 22]. Salvage surgery can be offered in many recurrent cases [16]. Penile preservation rates are reported to be better in brachytherapy: 50–66% for external radiotherapy vs. 75–86% for brachytherapy [21, 22].

Radiation therapy carries a high rate of acute and chronic complications, that in severe cases terminate treatment or lead to penile amputation. For external radiotherapy and brachytherapy, the following complication rates are reported: radiation necrosis – 1–8% and 6–23%, urethral strictures – 3–45% and 9–45% [21, 22] (Fig. 5.1).

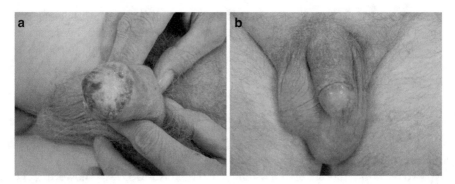

Fig. 5.1 Post-radiotherapy complications. (**a**) Glans necrosis. (**b**) Telangiectasia and chronic ulceration

Other radiation reactions are also observed: meatal stenosis (6,6–40%), dysuria (5,3%), pain during intercourse (2,6%), fibrosis, chronic ulceration, pigmentation and telangiectasia [1, 21, 22] (Fig. 5.1).

An alternative type of brachytherapy: Surface mould plesiotherapy is a technique developed for treatment of superficial tumours (Tis, T1a or T1b). An appliance containing iridium wire sources is worn around the penis for several hours daily for up to 1 week. This technique is not recommended for tumours invading the corpus spongiosum or lesions thicker than 5 mm. Up to 79% of complete response was reported primarily, but in a longer term almost 45% of patients required salvage surgery [23].

Another important limitation of radiotherapy is that associated skin reactions can make diagnosis of recurrence challenging.

Penile-Sparing Surgical Techniques

Moh's Micrographic Surgery (MMC)

Indication: PeIN and pT1a penile cancer.

The technique historically developed for skin tumours has been adopted to superficial penile cancers. It relies on geometric conical/cross-sectional excisions of subsequent layers of tissue with synchronous frozen sections aiming to achieve negative resection margin. This option allows precise excision of tumour with maximal tissue preservation. In long-term observation (over 3 years), local recurrence for PeIN is 5%, while for penile squamous cell cancer (SCC), it varies between 0% to 32% [24, 25]. Nodal recurrences were reported in 8% of cases [24, 25]. Most local recurrences can be further treated with MMC or penile-preserving techniques; however, cancer specific death was reported [24, 25]. Mohs surgery provides best outcomes in very selected patients with small, low-grade tumours without urethral involvement [24, 25]. Mohs technique is time-consuming, technically demanding and it requires trained team of specialists. For these reasons, it was not popularised outside several specialised centres. One of the most common complications is meatal stenosis (6–16%) [24, 25].

Laser Therapy

Indication: PeIN and pT1a penile cancer.

Two types of lasers are used most often: CO_2 and Nd-YAG laser; however, KTP and argon lasers were also adopted in penile cancer treatment [1]. Laser treatment can be performed in a form of dissection (mostly carbon dioxide (CO_2) laser) or ablation (mostly Nd-YAG laser). Application of acetic acid before the treatment is advised for accurate examination and surgery planning [26, 27]. Primary laser treatment is usually combined with circumcision for safety and hygiene improvement [26, 27]. Treatment is usually well tolerated with average healing time of 6 weeks. Long-term series report high aesthetic satisfaction rate reaching 80–100% and high proportion (up to 60%) of sexual function preservation [26, 27] . A large series reported 5 and 10 year recurrence rate of 14.1% and 17.5%, respectively [27]. All patients were managed with further laser therapy, radiotherapy or amputation, with the latter required in 2.9% at 5 years and 5.5% at 10 years [27].

Overall, with different types of lasers, various stages of the treated disease (PeIN – invasive malignancies) and treatment protocols the recurrence rates range from 10% to 48% [26, 28].

One needs to remember that thermal tissue damage may compromise pathologic evaluation thus hampering tumour staging. On the other hand, taking a biopsy prior to laser treatment carries the risk of under-staging.

Post-operative bleeding, urethral stenosis and preputial adhesions to the coronal sulcus were reported in a small proportion of patients (<1%, <1% and <3% of cases) [27]. With careful patient selection and meticulous follow-up in laser-experienced centres, this modality offers good results with minimal morbidity.

Circumcision

Indication: PeIN and pT1 tumours confined to prepuce.

Circumcision is one of the most common procedures performed for penile precancerous and cancerous lesions. Radical circumcision is mainstay of treatment for tumours confined to prepuce, provided that negative margins are achieved. Acetowhite reaction of dysplastic and neoplastic lesions to 5% acetic acid application can be useful to confirm complete excision or plan further treatment. It is particularly helpful in HPV-related tumours, but shows limitations due to low specificity and false positivity in differentiation in chronic inflammatory conditions [29]. Two options are possible if pre-cancer is confirmed at the mucosal excision margin: either wide local excision of disease involving glans or/and shaft or topical chemotherapy applied once the circumcision scar has healed [4].

Circumcision is advised as supplementary treatment to topical chemotherapy, laser treatment and treatment of glandular tumours [1, 26, 27]. It also has preventive role by removing the chronic inflammatory promoting milieu and minimising risk of progression to malignant lesions. In addition, it aids clinical examination that is crucial to follow-up strategies.

Glans Resurfacing

Indication: PeIN and pT1 penile cancer.

This technique includes excision of epithelial and subepithelial glans tissue followed by replacement with partial thickness skin graft. It was primarily developed by Bracka for treatment of extensive cases of lichen sclerosus [30]. It was later adapted for the treatment of premalignant lesions and superficial tumours (Tis, Ta up to pT1a) of the glans [31–33]. It can be offered in cases of in situ malignancy: to individuals with extensive changes, patients who failed topical treatment, do not accept it or are unlikely to follow surveillance protocol afterwards. In cases of localised disease, if less than 50% of the glans is involved partial glans resurfacing is a feasible option [32].

After placing a tourniquet, glans epithelial and subepithelial tissue is excised in four quadrants starting with incision around the meatal opening down to the retrocoronal sulcus. In non-circumcised patients, circumcision is part of the procedure. In selected cases, deep spongiosal biopsy may be sent for frozen section analysis to confirm radical resection. The specimen is oriented for accurate histopathology assessment. Penile shaft skin is then approximated below the coronal sulcus and the glans covered with split thickness skin graft (STSG). Fine absorbable sutures are used to secure the graft to the coronal and urethral margin. Quilting sutures are placed to stabilise the graft. (Fig. 5.2) A urethral catheter is inserted, compressive dressing applied, and bed rest is advised for 48 hours post-operatively. The catheter is removed with the securing dressing on fifth post-operative day [31, 32]. Eight weeks later, the graft is fully healed (Fig. 5.2).

Partial glans resurfacing relies on the same principle of epithelial and subepithelial tissue excision and STSG coverage, but only in the involved part of the glans. This allows to preserve a proportion of natural glans mucosa and potentially better glans sensation in comparison to complete glans resurfacing. It provides aesthetically pleasing results (Fig. 5.3). Where excision margins are difficult to assess macroscopically, acetic acid can be helpful to guide limits of the excision. The risk of incomplete excision and positive margin is however higher in comparison to complete glans resurfacing, and patients need to be adequately informed [32]. Results validate this option as the local recurrence rate is low, and it should not compromise

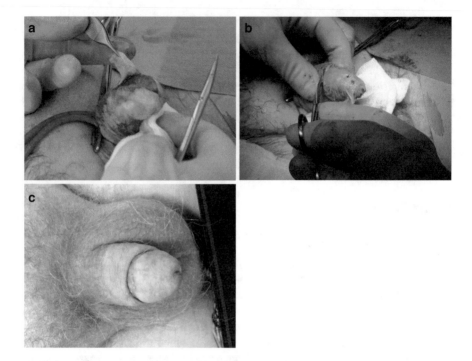

Fig. 5.2 Total glans resurfacing for penile cancer. (**a**) The glans epithelium and sub-epithelium are excised in quadrants, starting from the urethral meatal margin towards the coronal sulcus. (**b**) The glans penis is covered by partial thickness skin graft. (**c**) Post-operative appearance following total glans resurfacing

patients' prognosis. If needed, radical treatment is achieved by further penile-preserving techniques such as glans resurfacing or glansectomy with STSG reconstruction [32].

Glans resurfacing provides excellent aesthetic and functional outcomes without compromise to oncological results [31–35]. There is no, or only minimal, risk of intraoperative and post-operative complications such as compromised graft take and infection [31–35]. The procedure provides definitive histopathology results, thus enabling further follow-up planning and treatment if needed. In up to 20% of patients undergoing glans resurfacing for penile intraepithelial neoplasia (PeIN), invasive malignancy is diagnosed despite previous incisional biopsies confirming PeIN only [32]. Preoperative biopsy was shown to be accurate in 34% of patients [36]. This emphasizes the importance of an accurate histopathology assessment, meticulous follow-up and explains why conservative treatment options can underestimate the disease and result in recurrence [17].

Up to 28% of patients treated with glans resurfacing required further surgery [32], with local recurrence rate of 0–4% for PeIN [31, 32, 35] and 0–11.5% for pT1a [32–36]. No nodal recurrences and no influence on survival were reported at 16–38 months of mean follow-up [32–35].

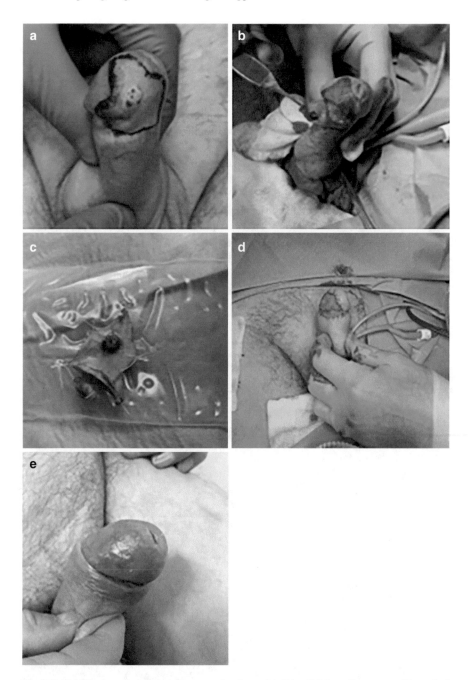

Fig. 5.3 Partial glans resurfacing for cutaneous horn. (**a**) Superficial penile cancer with marked excision limits. (**b**) Removal of epithelial and subepithelial tissues with cancerous lesion. (**c**) Specimen – oriented for histopathology assessment. (**d**) Split thickness skin graft covering glans and coronal sulcus. (**e**) 8 weeks post-surgery – healed graft

Glansectomy

Indication: T1 to T2 penile cancer.

Complete removal of the glans spongiosum separated from cavernosal heads for tumours involving the glans was primarily described by Austoni [37]. This option is feasible for T2 tumours and high-grade T1 tumours. In cases of small lesions occupying part of the glans, the technique can be modified to wide local excision (WLE) and partial glansectomy.

Glansectomy is usually performed under regional/general anaesthetic and local block. A proximal incision below the level of the coronal sulcus is made, and the plane between glans and corporal tips is developed, below or above the Buck's fascia depending on tumour extent [38]. The glans spongiosum is resected of the cavernosal tips, and the urethra is transected as a last element of the specimen. (Fig. 5.4) In selected cases, frozen section is helpful to confirm complete excision at the level of urethral and/or corporal margin [10, 16]. The urethra is positioned centrally within the cavernosal tips to provide better voiding parameters and cosmesis. Penile shaft skin is secured circumferentially to the distal shaft forming a new corona. The remaining exposed surface of the corpora cavernosa is covered with STSG from the

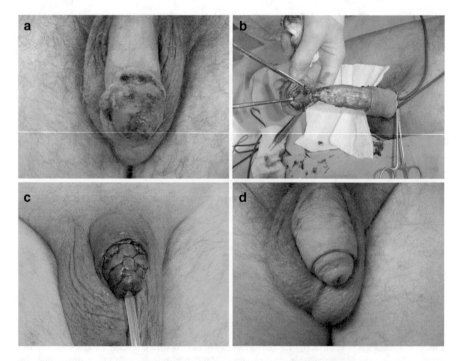

Fig. 5.4 Glansectomy. (**a**) Penile cancer at the glans penis. (**b**) Glansectomy in progress – glans dissected off corporal tips, before division of urethra. (**c**) Creation of a neoglans using partial thickness skin graft reconstruction. (**d**) Post-operative appearance of the healed neoglans

thigh analogous to glans resurfacing, forming the neoglans. Post-operative dressing and management are identical to glans resurfacing surgery with 48 hours bed rest, stabilising dressing and catheter left for 5 days.

Partial glansectomy and wide local excision are amenable for smaller tumours involving less than half of the glans/leaving residual epithelium [28]. (Fig. 5.5) An involved part of the glans is removed with macroscopically preserved margins. The glans can be primarily closed in the case of small lesions, but larger defects can leave a deformed glans and should be reconstructed with penile skin flaps, STSG or full thickness penile shaft skin graft for good aesthetic outcome. This option is dedicated to patients willing to obey strict follow-up protocol, as the technique leaves a higher potential for recurrence in comparison to glansectomy [16]. Early detection of local recurrence still leaves an option for a radical treatment through salvage total glansectomy or partial penectomy providing good oncological outcomes [28, 39–41].

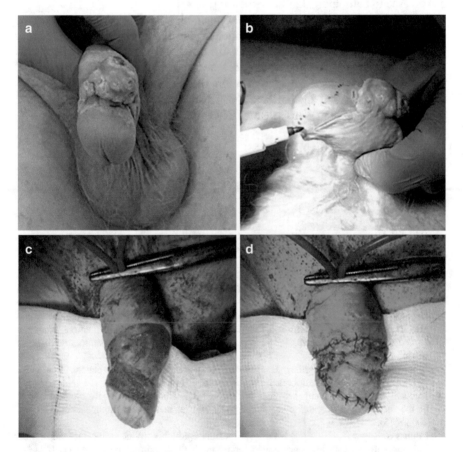

Fig. 5.5 Partial glansectomy. (**a**) Tumour of the coronal sulcus involving glans and inner prepuce. (**b**) Excision limits marked on the skin. (**c**) Tumour excised with superficial glans epithelium and circumcision. (**d**) Defect covered with split thickness skin graft

Glansectomy offers excellent oncologic results with local recurrence rate of 0–3% [16, 42] for partial glansectomy and 0–16% for glansectomy [9, 10, 12, 16, 35, 38–40, 43–46] with no implications on cancer-specific survival in most of the studies and disease-free survival of 90%–100% during a mean 10–42 months follow-up period [10, 16, 38–40, 42, 45]. A recent study suggests, however, that local recurrence, lympho-vascular invasion and clinical nodal status are identified as predictors of compromised cancer-specific survival [12]. It is likely a result of an aggressive disease rather than an incomplete tumour excision, which highlights importance of appropriate patient selection.

Further treatment can be offered immediately in cases of a positive surgical margin or local recurrence. The latter should trigger complete restaging in patients after OSS [16, 41]. Features such as perineural invasion, penile intraepithelial neoplasia, positive definitive margins, lympho-vascular invasion, high-grade SCC and pT3 stage have been identified as risk factors for local recurrence after glansectomy and can be used to tailor individual surveillance [12, 47].

A low risk of complications has been reported, including partial graft loss or contraction (requiring surgical intervention in up to 9% of patients), infection, meatal stenosis and compromised sensation [9, 10, 16, 28, 35, 38, 39, 46]. Few studies addressed sexual function after glansectomy; the available data suggests most of the patients who were sexually active before the surgery remain active after treatment [10, 39, 42, 44, 46] and preserve their erectile, orgasmic and ejaculatory functions, with a reduction in glans sensitivity [43–45].

References

1. Hakenberg OW, Compérat E, Minhas S, et al. EAU guidelines on penile cancer. EAU Guidel. 2020.
2. Oertell J, Ocampos S, Boggino H, Codas R. Epidemiologic profile, sexual history, pathologic features, and human papillomavirus status of 103 patients with penile carcinoma. World J Urol. 2013;31(4):861–7. https://doi.org/10.1007/s00345-011-0802-0.
3. Bayles AC, Sethia KK. The impact of improving outcomes guidance on the management and outcomes of patients with. Ann R Coll Surg Engl. 2010;92:44–5. https://doi.org/10.1308/003588410X12518836439047.
4. Hegarty PK, Shabbir M, Hughes B, et al. Penile preserving surgery and surgical strategies to maximize penile form and function in penile cancer: recommendations from the United Kingdom experience. World J Urol. 2009;27(2):179–87. https://doi.org/10.1007/s00345-008-0312-x.
5. Branney P, Witty K, Eardley I. Patients ' experiences of penile cancer. Eur Urol. 2011;59(6):959–61. https://doi.org/10.1016/j.eururo.2011.02.009.
6. Agrawal A, Pai D, Ananthakrishnan N, Smile SR, Ratnakar C. The histological extent of the local spread of carcinoma of the penis and its therapeutic implications. BJU Int. 2000;85(3):299–301.
7. Minhas S, Kayes O, Hegarty P, Kumar P, Freeman A, Ralph D. What surgical resection margins are required to achieve oncological control in men with primary penile cancer? BJU Int. 2005;96(7):2–5. https://doi.org/10.1111/j.1464-410X.2005.05769.x.

8. Hoffman MA, Renshaw AA, Loughlin KR. Squamous cell carcinoma of the penis and microscopic pathologic margins: how much margin is needed for local cure? Cancer. 1999;85(7):1565–8.
9. Philippou P, Shabbir M, Malone P, et al. Conservative surgery for squamous cell carcinoma of the penis: resection margins and long-term oncological control. J Urol. 2012;188(3):803–8. https://doi.org/10.1016/j.juro.2012.05.012.
10. Smith Y, Hadway P, Biedrzycki O, Perry MJA, Corbishley C, Watkin NA. Reconstructive surgery for invasive squamous carcinoma of the Glans penis. Eur Urol. 2007;52:1179–85. https://doi.org/10.1016/j.eururo.2007.02.038.
11. Sri D, Sujenthiran A, Lam W, Minter J, Tinwell BE, Corbishley CM, Yap T, Sharma DM, Ayres BEWN. A study into the association between local recurrence rates and surgical resection margins in organ-sparing surgery for penile squamous cell cancer. BJU Int. 2018;122(4):576–82. https://doi.org/10.1111/bju.14222.
12. Roussel E, Peeters E, Vanthoor J, Bozzini G, Muneer A, Ayres B, Sri D, Watkin N, Bhattar R, Parnham A, Sangar V, Lau M, Joice G, Bivalacqua TJ, Chipollini J, Spiess PE, Hatzichristodoulou G, de Vries L, Brouwer OAM. Predictors of local recurrence and its impact on survival after glansectomy for penile cancer: time to challenge the dogma? BJU Int. 2020;127(5):606–13. https://doi.org/10.1111/bju.15297.
13. Djajadiningrat RS, Van Werkhoven E, Meinhardt W, et al. Penile sparing surgery for penile cancer–does it affect survival? J Urol. 2014;192(1):120–6. https://doi.org/10.1016/j.juro.2013.12.038.
14. Leijte JAP, Kirrander P, Antonini N, Windahl T, Horenblas S. Recurrence patterns of squamous cell carcinoma of the penis: recommendations for follow-up based on a two-centre analysis of 700 patients. Eur Urol. 2008;54:161–9. https://doi.org/10.1016/j.eururo.2008.04.016.
15. Martins FE, Rodrigues RN, Lopez TM. Organ-preserving surgery for penile carcinoma. Adv Urol. 2008;4. https://doi.org/10.1155/2008/634216
16. Pietrzak P, Corbishley C, Watkin N. Organ-sparing surgery for invasive penile cancer: early follow-up data. BJU Int. 2004;94:1253–7. https://doi.org/10.1111/j.1464-410X.2004.05153.x.
17. Alnajjar HM, Lam W, Bolgeri M, Rees RW, Perry MJA, Watkin NA. Treatment of carcinoma in situ of the Glans penis with topical chemotherapy agents. Eur Urol. 2012;62:923–8.
18. Hajiran A, Zemp L, Aydin AM, et al. Topical chemotherapy for penile carcinoma in situ: contemporary outcomes and reported toxicity. Urol Oncol. 2020;39(1). https://doi.org/10.1016/j.urolonc.2020.09.021
19. Porter WM, Francis N, Hawkins D, Dinneen M, Bunker CB. Clinical and Laboratory Investigations Penile intraepithelial neoplasia: clinical spectrum and treatment of 35 cases. Br J Dermatol. 2002;147(6):1159–65.
20. Kravvas G, Ge L, Ng J, et al. The management of penile intraepithelial neoplasia (PeIN): clinical and histological features and treatment of 345 patients and a review of the literature. J Dermatolog Treat. 2020;8(6):1–16. https://doi.org/10.1080/09546634.2020.1800574.
21. Azrif M, Logue JP, Swindell R, Cowan RA, Wylie JP, Livsey JE. External-beam radiotherapy in T1-2 N0 penile carcinoma. Clin Oncol. 2006;18(4):320–5. https://doi.org/10.1016/j.clon.2006.01.004.
22. Crook JUMC, Jezioranski JOHNJ, Math MM, Grimard LAG, Esche BEE, Pond GP. Penile brachytherapy: results for 49 patients. Int J Radiat Oncol. 2005;62(2):460–7. https://doi.org/10.1016/j.ijrobp.2004.10.016.
23. Korzeniowski MA, Crook JM. Contemporary role of radiotherapy in the management of penile cancer. Transl Androl Urol. 2017;6(5):855–67. https://doi.org/10.21037/tau.2017.07.02
24. Machan M, Brodland D, Zitelli J. Penile squamous cell carcinoma: penis-preserving treatment with Mohs micrographic surgery. Dermatol Surg. 2016;42(8):936–44. https://doi.org/10.1097/DSS.0000000000000795.
25. Shindel AW, Mann MW, Lev RY, et al. Mohs micrographic surgery for penile cancer: management and long-term follow up. J Urol. 2007;178(November):1980–5. https://doi.org/10.1016/j.juro.2007.07.039.

26. Schlenker B, Tilki D, Seitz M, et al. Organ-preserving neodymium-yttrium-aluminium-garnet laser therapy for penile carcinoma: a long-term follow-up. BJU Int. 2010;106(6):786–90. https://doi.org/10.1111/j.1464-410X.2009.09188.x.
27. Bandieramonte G, Colecchia M, Mariani L, et al. Peniscopically controlled CO 2 laser excision for conservative treatment of in situ and T1 penile carcinoma: report on 224 patients. Eur Urol. 2008;54(4):875–84. https://doi.org/10.1016/j.eururo.2008.01.019.
28. Lont AP, Gallee MPW, Meinhardt W, Van Tinteren H, Horenblas S. Penis conserving treatment for T1 and T2 penile carcinoma: clinical implications of a local recurrence. J Urol. 2006;176(August):575–80. https://doi.org/10.1016/j.juro.2006.03.063.
29. Wikstrom A, Hedblad M, Johansson B, Kalantari M, Syrjanen S, Lindberg M. The acetic acid test in evaluation of subclinical genital papillomavirus infection: a comparative study on penoscopy , histopathology , virology and scanning electron microscopy findings. Genitourin Med. 1992;68(2):90–9.
30. Depasquale I, Park AJ, Bracka A. The treatment of balanitis xerotica obliterans. BJU Int. 2000;86:459–65. https://doi.org/10.4103/0970-0358.81455.
31. Hadway P, Corbishley CM, Watkin NA. Total glans resurfacing for premalignant lesions of the penis: initial outcome data. BJU Int. 2006;98:532–6. https://doi.org/10.1111/j.1464-410X .2006.06368.x.
32. Shabbir M, Muneer A, Kalsi J, et al. Glans resurfacing for the treatment of carcinoma in situ of the penis: surgical technique and outcomes. Eur Urol. 2011;59(1):142–7. https://doi. org/10.1016/j.eururo.2010.09.039.
33. Kelly FO, Lonergan P, Lundon D, et al. A prospective study of total glans resurfacing in localised penile cancer to maximise oncological and functional outcomes within a tertiary referral network. J Urol. 2017;197:1258–63. https://doi.org/10.1016/j.juro.2016.12.089.
34. Falcone M, Preto M, Oderda M, et al. Reconstructive urology management of superficial penile analysis in a tertiary referral center. Urology. 2020;145:281–6. https://doi.org/10.1016/j. urology.2020.06.066.
35. Håkansson ULF, Kirrander P, Uvelius B, Baseckas G, Torbrand C. Organ-sparing reconstructive surgery in penile cancer: initial experiences at two Swedish referral centres. Scand J Urol. 2015;49:149–54. https://doi.org/10.3109/21681805.2014.955822.
36. Ayres B, Lam W, Al-najjar H, Corbishley C, Perry M, Watkin N. Oncological outcomes of glans resurfacing in the treatment of selected superficially invasive penile cancers. J Urol. 2012;187(4):e306. https://doi.org/10.1016/j.juro.2012.02.832.
37. Austoni E, Fenice O, Kartalas Goumas Y, Colombo F, Mantovani FPE. New trends in the surgical treatment of penile carcinoma. Arch Ital Urol Androl. 1996;68:163–8.
38. Parnham AS, Albersen M, Sahdev V, et al. Glansectomy and Split-thickness skin graft for penile cancer. Eur Urol. 2016;73(2):284–9. https://doi.org/10.1016/j.eururo.2016.09.048.
39. Kane HFO, Pahuja A, Ho KJ, Thwaini A, Nambirajan T, Keane P. Outcome of Glansectomy and skin grafting in the management of penile cancer. Adv Urol. 2011;4(4):1–4. https://doi. org/10.1155/2011/240824.
40. Tang ADH, Yan S, Ottenhof SR, et al. Department of Urological Oncology , Netherlands Cancer Institute , Amsterdam, the Corresponding Author: Department of Genitourinary Oncology. Urology. 2017;109:140–4. https://doi.org/10.1016/j.urology.2017.08.004.
41. Baumgarten A, Chipollini J, Yan S, et al. Penile sparing surgery for penile cancer: a multicenter international retrospective cohort. J Urol. 2018;199(5):1233–7. https://doi.org/10.1016/j. juro.2017.10.045.
42. Brown CT, Minhas S, Ralph DJ. Conservative surgery for penile cancer: subtotal glans excision without grafting. BJU Int. 2005;96(6):911–2. https://doi.org/10.1111/j.1464-410X.2005. 05751.x.
43. Morelli G, Pagni R, Mariani C, Campo G, Minervini R, Minervini A. Glansectomy with split-thickness skin graft for the treatment of penile carcinoma. Int J Impot Res. 2009;02:311–4. https://doi.org/10.1038/ijir.2009.17.

44. Palminteri E, Berdondini E, Lazzeri M, et al. Resurfacing and reconstruction of the Glans penis. Eur Urol. 2007;52:893–900. https://doi.org/10.1016/j.eururo.2007.01.047.
45. Gulino G, Sasso F, Falabella R, Bassi PF. Distal urethral reconstruction of the Glans for penile carcinoma: results of a novel technique at 1-year of followup. J Urol. 2007;178(3):941–4. https://doi.org/10.1016/j.juro.2007.05.059.
46. Beech BB, Chapman DW, Rourke KF. Clinical outcomes of glansectomy with split-thickness skin graft reconstruction for localized penile cancer. Can Urol Assoc J. 2020;14(10):1–10.
47. Albersen M, Ph D, Parnham A, et al. Predictive factors for local recurrence after glansectomy and neoglans reconstruction for penile squamous cell carcinoma. Urol Oncol. 2017;36(4):141–6. https://doi.org/10.1016/j.urolonc.2017.07.025.
48. Brierley JD, Gospodarowicz MK, Wittekind C. TNM classification of malignant tumours. 8th ed. John Wiley & Sons, Ltd.; 2017. https://www.wiley.com/en-ad/TNM+Classification+of+Malignant+Tumours%2C+8th+Edition-p-9781119263562.

Chapter 6
Management of Primary Penile Tumours: Partial and Total Penectomy

Karl H. Pang, Hussain M. Alnajjar, and Asif Muneer

Introduction

Penile cancer (PCa) is a rare cancer that predominantly arises from the preputial skin and glans of the penis. PCa mostly affects men of advanced age with a peak incidence in the sixth decade. Localised and advanced PCa and their treatment can have significant physical and psychosexual effects and, therefore, impact on the quality of life of cancer survivors.

This chapter covers the surgical techniques of partial and total penectomy for primary PCa. Other aspects of PCa including aetio-pathogenesis and organ-sparing surgery are covered elsewhere in this book.

K. H. Pang
Academic Urology Unit, University of Sheffield, Sheffield, UK

Section of Andrology, Pyrah Department of Urology, St James' Hospital, The Leeds Teaching Hospitals NHS Trust, Leeds, UK
e-mail: karl.pang@nhs.net

H. M. Alnajjar
Institute of Andrology and UCL Male Genital Cancer Centre, University College London Hospitals NHS Foundation Trust, London, UK
e-mail: hussain.alnajjar@nhs.net

A. Muneer (✉)
Institute of Andrology and UCL Male Genital Cancer Centre, University College London Hospitals NHS Foundation Trust, London, UK

Division of Surgery and Interventional Science, University College London, London, UK

NIHR Biomedical Research Centre University College London Hospitals, London, UK
e-mail: asif.muneer@nhs.net

Surgical Treatment of Penile Cancer

The extent of tumour invasion will determine the surgical treatment option. Although oncological control with tumour removal and clear margins is the aim of cancer surgery, PCa also requires attention to preservation of function, including the ability to have penetrative sexual intercourse and voiding standing up. Therefore, penile-preserving procedures have been the mainstay of treatment for the past three decades, and partial and total penectomy is reserved for more extensive lesions invading into the corpus cavernosum. Penile MRI is used to stage the disease, and more importantly, to check the degree of invasion into the corpora (cT2 – corpus spongiosum, cT3 – corpus cavernosum invasion).

Premalignant disease referred to as penile intraepithelial neoplasia (PeIN) can be managed using topical chemotherapy (5-FU) or immunotherapy (Imiquimod). Where these options fail, glans resurfacing can be offered. Ta, T1a (no lymphovascular invasion) disease can be managed with wide local excision with circumcision, laser ablation with circumcision or glans resurfacing [1, 2].

T1b (lymphovascular invasion) and T2 disease can be managed with wide local excision or for more extensive lesions – a glansectomy and split skin graft. However, when the disease invades the corpus cavernosum (T3) with or without involvement of the urethra, partial penectomy with reconstruction can be offered. In some T3 cases where preserving the penis is not possible, a total penectomy with formation of a perineal urethrostomy is required [1, 2]. Often preoperative imaging detects disease more proximally in the crura in which case a radical penectomy is indicated.

Partial Penectomy

Men with disease involving the distal corpus cavernosum and urethra require a partial penectomy, if there is an adequate stump length of at least 5 cm to maintain functional outcomes [1, 3–5]. Those without a 5 cm stump length or where there is proximal disease are best managed with a total penectomy and formation of a perineal urethrostomy.

There is no clear consensus as to the acceptable clear surgical margins. Historically, a 2 cm excision margin was the standard of care; however, it is now evident that much smaller margins, especially with organ-sparing surgery do not affect long-term oncological outcomes [6]. The EAU guidelines [1] suggest that 3–5 mm can be considered a safe margin. A grade-based differentiated approach can also be used, with 3 mm for grade 1, 5 mm for grade 2 and 8 mm for grade 3 [1]. An analysis of 179 men with invasive PCa treated with organ-sparing surgery at a single tertiary centre demonstrated a 5-year local recurrence-free rate of 86.3%. The authors concluded that penile-preserving surgery is oncologically safe, and a surgical excision margin of even less than 5 mm is adequate [7]. The shift towards smaller margins has improved both functional and cosmetic outcomes without compromising oncological outcomes [1, 3, 6, 7].

Surgical Technique

There are a number of techniques in performing a partial penectomy.

Patient Preparation

The patient is placed in the supine position and following the administration of perioperative antibiotics, a local anaesthetic penile block is performed.

A circumferential incision is made on the penile shaft skin proximal to the tumour down to the level of Buck's fascia (Fig. 6.1a). The dorsal neurovascular bundle is identified, mobilised and ligated. A tourniquet is applied to the base of the penis before the distal corpora and urethra are transected. The corpus cavernosum is oversewn with 3–0 absorbable sutures, and approximately 1 cm of urethral length is preserved and spatulated ventrally (Fig. 6.1b–d). Further biopsies from the proximal corporal margin and urethra can be sent for frozen-section analysis in order to ensure that the margins are free of tumour. The penile shaft skin is mobilised to prevent later retraction and shortening, and the spatulated urethra is sutured to the penile shaft skin. Alternatively, a more rounded neoglans can be reconstructed from the corpora, and a split thickness skin graft (SSG, ~0.012–0.016 inch) harvested from the anterior thigh using a dermatome is then quilted to the denuded corporal heads with 5–0 absorbable sutures. A dressing is sutured to the neoglans to prevent any disruption to the graft. A urethral catheter is placed, and the dressings are removed between 7 to 10 days [8, 9].

Other Surgical Aspects

With the standard technique, the urethral meatus is commonly sited in an abnormal ventral position, with an associated risk of meatal stenosis. A urethral centralisation (UCAPP) technique has been described, which allows the restoration of the meatus to the tip of the neoglans, improving the overall cosmetic appearance and reducing the psychological morbidity (Fig. 6.1d). The urethra is mobilised to allow the formation of a urethrostomy at the tip of the penis. The shaft skin is sutured 2 cm from the tip leaving the corporal heads exposed. A split thickness skin graft is quilted to create a neoglans [10].

An alternative to 'quilting' the skin graft onto the neoglans is the tie-over method (TODGA technique), which fixes a proflavine-soaked gauze to the skin graft allowing immediate patient mobilisation and discharge home with a catheter (Fig. 6.1e). Hospital stay is reduced, and excellent cosmetic results (Fig. 6.1f) are achieved with a high percentage of graft uptake [11].

Penile lengthening manoeuvres can also be performed at the same time of partial penectomy or at a later date. An extra 2–3 cm can be gained by degloving the penis and dividing the penile suspensory ligaments (Fig. 6.2). Penile length extension can also be achieved by surgically releasing an existing penoscrotal web at the ventral aspect via a V-Y-plasty or Z-plasty [5].

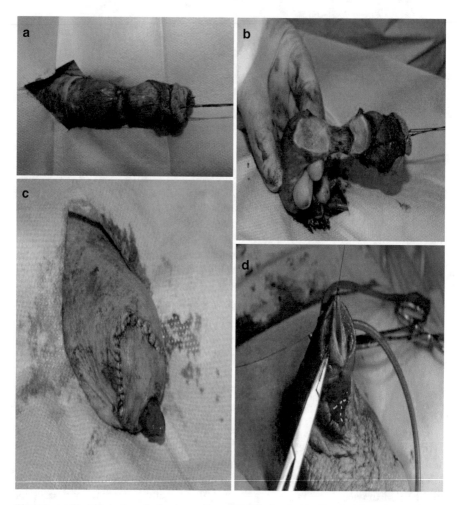

Fig. 6.1 (**a**) The skin and penile fascia are dissected to the level of Buck's fascia and the neurovascular bundle ligated. (**b**) The penis is transected leaving the urethra protruding by 1.5 cm. (**c**) Closure of the penile skin showing the position of the neourethra, which is then sutured to the penile skin. (**d**) Partial penectomy with urethral centralization where the corpora are wrapped around the urethra rather than being oversewn. (**e**) TODGA dressing applied after urethral centralization and grafting of the neoglans. (**f**) Post-operative result following partial penectomy and urethral centralization

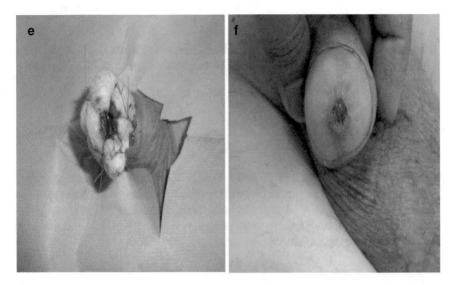

Fig. 6.1 (continued)

Fig. 6.2 Division of the suspensory ligament allows penile mobilization in order to gain additional length

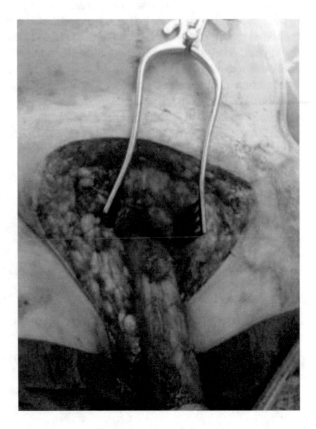

Post-Operative Complications

The main complications related to partial penectomy is meatal stenosis and graft failure. Meatal stenosis can be minimised by ensuring adequate mobilisation of the urethra and spatulation.

Total Penectomy

Total penectomy is indicated in T3 or T4 stage PCa, if a functional residual stump is not possible. Radical penectomy involves excising the penis with removal of the corporal body down to the level of the pubic bone. Following the excision of the penis, the urethra is brought through the perineum to form a perineal urethrostomy, therefore requiring men to sit down to void.

Surgical Technique

The patient is positioned in the lithotomy position and peri-operative antibiotics are administered. An elliptical incision is marked around the penis that incorporates the upper scrotal skin. The scrotal skin and superficial fascia are incised. The penis is mobilised proximally, and the deep dorsal vein and neurovascular bundle is ligated and divided. The suspensory ligament is divided and the dissection continues proximally down to the pubic bone where the crura are transected and plicated. The urethra is transected and spatulated ventrally, and a separate inverted U or λ shaped incision is performed in the perineum (Fig. 6.3). The urethra is brought out and the spatulated ventral end is sutured to the apex of the inverted U incision with 4–0 vicryl sutures. A drain is left in the pubic area to reduce the formation of haematoma, and a urethral catheter is placed for 7 days [9].

Fig. 6.3 Incision (inverted U or λ) utilized to form a perineal urethrostomy

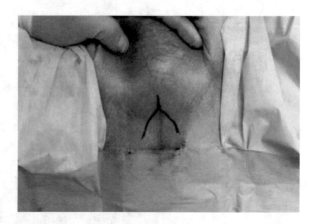

Post-Operative Complications

Stenosis of the perineal urethrostomy is a complication that may require revision surgery. The stenosis can be avoided by ensuring that the inverted U at the perineum has a fairly obtuse angle at the apex and that the ventral urethral spatulation is of an adequate length.

Phallic Reconstruction

Phallic reconstruction is an option to create a penis that permits resumption of sexual activity in previous sexually active men. Surgical reconstructive techniques provide good oncological outcomes whilst minimising emasculation. Free tissue flaps are commonly harvested from the forearm on the radial artery supply, but alternative donor sites include the anterolateral thigh, the scapula or latissimus dorsi, fibula, and local rotational flaps from the abdomen, groin and thigh. A penile prosthesis placed within the neophallus in a staged procedure is often needed to provide an enhanced phallic rigidity [5, 12, 13]. When performing a total penectomy, the remaining corpora can house the rear tips of a delayed penile prosthesis. Therefore, in the younger age group who are more likely to undergo a reconstruction, where possible the urethral length should be preserved even if it involves bringing the urethra out onto the anterior scrotal wall rather than a perineal urethrostomy.

A retrospective review of 15 patients who underwent radial-artery free flap provided good cosmetic and functional outcomes. Almost all patients ($n = 14$, 93.3%) were able to void while standing, seven (46.7%) patients had a penile prosthesis inserted and five were engaged in sexual intercourse at a median follow-up of 20 months [14].

Oncological Outcome

The oncological outcome following a diagnosis of PCa depends on the histology, grade and TNM stage. Lymph node staging and management of lymph node-positive disease, as well as metastatic disease are covered elsewhere.

A series of 32 partial penectomies reported one local recurrence (3.1%) and 12 deaths (37.5%) at a median follow-up of 22 months. The 3-year overall survival rate was 56% [15].

In a retrospective analysis of 700 patients with penile SCC in the Netherlands, 285 men underwent partial or total penectomy and 415 men underwent penile-preserving treatment. The median follow-up was 60.6 months. Recurrence occurred in less men in the amputation group ($n = 15$, 5.3%) compared with those who had penile-preserving procedures ($n = 115$, 27.7%). The 5-year disease-specific survival was 92% after a local recurrence, and 32.7% after a regional recurrence [16].

A contemporary North American series on penile surgery for 4238 men with pT1–2 PCa showed that the 5-year and 10-year overall survival rates were 85% and 72% for partial penectomy, respectively, and 79% and 63% for total penectomy [17].

Functional Outcome and Quality of Life

The surgical treatment of PCa is disfiguring and will affect sexual life, psychosocial well-being [18, 19]. An early study by D'Ancona et al., which involved interviewing and surveying 14 men who underwent partial penectomy for PCa, showed that the overall sexual interest, satisfaction and frequency of sexual intercourse was unchanged or slightly decreased in nine men (64%). The masculine self-image and the relationship with their partners remained unchanged in all patients [20].

Romero et al. interviewed 18 men who underwent partial penectomy and reported that 55.6% had sufficient erectile function to allow sexual intercourse. However, 66.7% maintained the same frequency and level of sexual desire as before surgery, and 72.2% continued to have ejaculation and orgasm every time they had sexual stimulation or intercourse. Some reasons for not resuming sexual intercourse include a small penis size and the absence of the glans penis [21].

Keiffer et al. reported that 90 men after partial penectomy had more problems with orgasms, appearance concerns, life interference compared to those who underwent penile-sparing treatments. With regard to the IIEF-15 questionnaire, a significantly reduced score in the partial penectomy was only present in orgasmic function domain. A total of 83% of men experienced urinary incontinence after partial penectomy (43% with penile-sparing surgery), and 35% of men experienced incontinence and spraying of urine [22].

In more up-to-date data on sexual outcomes following partial penectomy, Sansalone et al. surveyed 15 men and found significant reduced scores in all five domains of the IIEF-15 questionnaire post-operatively. Treatment satisfaction was evaluated using the EDITS questionnaire, and nine (60%) men reported a high satisfaction rate [23].

A review of the US surveillance, Epidemiology, and End Results (SEER) database consisting of 6155 men with penile SCC revealed a suicide rate in 13 (0.2%) men. All patients that committed suicide had undergone surgical intervention. Despite the negative psychological effects on patients with PCa, suicide rates are among the lowest of all urological malignancies [24].

Conclusion

Penile cancer is a rare disease, but its presentation and subsequent surgical treatment may affect urinary and sexual function as well as psychosocial well-being. Following partial and total penectomy, reconstructive phalloplasty can be performed to allow sexual activity and maintain one's masculine self-image.

References

1. Hakenberg OW, Compérat E, Minhas S, Necchi A, Pretzel C, Watkin N. Penile Cancer [Internet]. EAU Guidel. 2021. Available from: https://uroweb.org/guideline/penile-cancer/.

2. Raskin Y, Vanthoor J, Milenkovic U, Muneer A, Albersen M. Organ-sparing surgical and nonsurgical modalities in primary penile cancer treatment. Curr Opin Urol. 2019; 29(2):156–64.
3. Thomas A, Necchi A, Muneer A, Tobias-Machado M, Tran ATH, Van Rompuy A-S, et al. Penile cancer. Nat Rev Dis Prim. 2021;7(1):11.
4. Ahmed ME, Khalil MI, Kamel MH, Karnes RJ, Spiess PE. Progress on Management of Penile Cancer in 2020. Curr Treat Options in Oncol. 2020;22(1):4.
5. Burnett AL. Penile preserving and reconstructive surgery in the management of penile cancer. Nat Rev Urol. 2016;13(5):249–57.
6. Minhas S, Kayes O, Hegarty P, Kumar P, Freeman A, Ralph D. What surgical resection margins are required to achieve oncological control in men with primary penile cancer? BJU Int. 2005;96(7):1040–3.
7. Philippou P, Shabbir M, Malone P, Nigam R, Muneer A, Ralph DJ, et al. Conservative surgery for squamous cell carcinoma of the penis: resection margins and long-term oncological control. J Urol. 2012;188(3):803–8.
8. Hadway P, Malone P, Muneer A. Management of penile cancer using penile-preserving techniques. In: Muneer A, Horenblas S, editors. Textbook of penile cancer. 2nd ed. London: Springer; 2016. p. 138–40.
9. Muneer A, Sangar V. Management of locally advanced and metastatic penile cancer. In: Muneer A, Horenblas S, editors. Textbook of penile cancer. 2nd ed. London: Springer; 2016. p. 146–51.
10. Kranz J, Parnham A, Albersen M, Sahdev V, Ziada M, Nigam R, et al. Urethral centralization and pseudo-glans formation after partial penectomy. Urologe A. 2017; 56(10):1293–7.
11. Malone PR, Thomas JS, Blick C. A tie-over dressing for graft application in distal penectomy and glans resurfacing: the TODGA technique. BJU Int. 2011;107(5):836–40.
12. Alnajjar HM, Randhawa K, Muneer A. Localized disease: types of reconstruction/plastic surgery techniques after glans resurfacing/glansectomy/partial/total penectomy. Curr Opin Urol. 2020;30(2):213–7.
13. Heston AL, Esmonde NO, Dugi DD, Berli JU. Phalloplasty: techniques and outcomes. Transl Androl Urol. 2019;8(3):254–65.
14. Garaffa G, Raheem AA, Christopher NA, Ralph DJ. Total phallic reconstruction after penile amputation for carcinoma. BJU Int. 2009;104(6):852–6.
15. Korets R, Koppie TM, Snyder ME, Russo P. Partial penectomy for patients with squamous cell carcinoma of the penis: the Memorial Sloan-Kettering experience. Ann Surg Oncol. 2007;14(12):3614–9.
16. Leijte JAP, Kirrander P, Antonini N, Windahl T, Horenblas S. Recurrence patterns of squamous cell carcinoma of the penis: recommendations for follow-up based on a two-centre analysis of 700 patients. Eur Urol. 2008;54(1):161–8.
17. Kamel MH, Tao J, Su J, Khalil MI, Bissada NK, Schurhamer B, et al. Survival outcomes of organ sparing surgery, partial penectomy, and total penectomy in pathological T1/T2 penile cancer: report from the National Cancer Data Base. Urol Oncol. 2018;36(2): 82.e7–15.
18. Audenet F, Sfakianos JP. Psychosocial impact of penile carcinoma. Transl Androl Urol. 2017;6(5):874–8.
19. Coba G, Patel T. Penile cancer: managing sexual dysfunction and improving quality of life after therapy. Curr Urol Rep. 2021;22(2):8.
20. D'Ancona CA, Botega NJ, De Moraes C, Lavoura NS, Santos JK, Rodrigues Netto N. Quality of life after partial penectomy for penile carcinoma. Urology. 1997;50(4):593–6.
21. Romero FR, dos Santos Romero KRP, de Mattos MAE, Garcia CRC, de Carvalho Fernandes R, Perez MDC. Sexual function after partial penectomy for penile cancer. Urology. 2005;66(6):1292–5.
22. Kieffer JM, Djajadiningrat RS, van Muilekom EAM, Graafland NM, Horenblas S, Aaronson NK. Quality of life for patients treated for penile cancer. J Urol. 2014;192(4):1105–10.

23. Sansalone S, Silvani M, Leonardi R, Vespasiani G, Iacovelli V. Sexual outcomes after par-
    tial penectomy for penile cancer: results from a multi-institutional study. Asian J Androl.
    2017;19(1):57–61.
24. Simpson WG, Klaassen Z, Jen RP, Hughes WM, Neal DE, Terris MK. Analysis of suicide
    risk in patients with penile cancer and review of the literature. Clin Genitourin Cancer.
    2018;16(2):e257–61.

Part III
Management of Inguinal and Pelvic Lymph Nodes

Chapter 7
In the Clinical Setting of Non-Palpable/ Non-Bulky Inguinal Nodes

Reza Nabavizadeh, Grace Lee, Katherine Bobrek, and Viraj A. Master

Introduction/Management Guidelines

The natural history and sequence of metastatic spread in penile carcinoma is well established in literature. From the primary site, cancer spreads to the superficial and deep inguinal lymph nodes, then to the pelvic nodes and distant sites. Inguinal nodal involvement may be bilateral due to extensive lymphatic networks at the base of the penis, while pelvic nodal involvement is usually ipsilateral [1]. Inguinal lymph node metastasis is a poor prognostic factor for survival in patients with penile cancer [2]. In a contemporary study, cancer-related mortality over a median follow-up time of 27 months was identified in 10.3%, 29.9%, 37.1%, and 47.2% of patients with N0, N1, N2, and N3 disease, respectively [3].

Management of patients in the clinical setting of non-palpable and non-bulky inguinal nodes (cN0) is challenging and can be controversial. First, clinical examination of the inguinal region may be limited due to body habitus or prior inguinal surgery [4]. In one study, physical exam findings were only 82% sensitive and 79% specific [5]. Additionally, up to 25% of patients with clinically negative nodes have occult metastatic disease on pathologic review of lymph nodes [6]. While this

R. Nabavizadeh · K. Bobrek
Department of Urology, Emory University, Atlanta, GA, USA
e-mail: reza.nabavizadeh@emory.edu; katya.bobrek@emory.edu

G. Lee
Rutgers Robert Wood Johnson Medical School, New Brunswick, NJ, USA

V. A. Master (✉)
Department of Urology, Emory University, Atlanta, GA, USA

Winship Cancer Institute, Emory University, Atlanta, GA, USA
e-mail: vmaster@emory.edu

© The Author(s), under exclusive license to Springer Nature Switzerland AG 2021   87
P. E. Spiess, A. Necchi (eds.), *Penile Carcinoma*,
https://doi.org/10.1007/978-3-030-82060-2_7

incidence is high, prophylactic ILND on all patients with penile cancer would imply overtreatment in majority of the patients. Inguinal lymph node dissection is traditionally associated with significant postoperative morbidity. The most common complications include lymphedema, wound infection, seroma formation, and skin-flap necrosis [7]. Gopman et al. reported a complication rate of 55.4%, of which 65.7% were minor and 34.3% major, and Stuiver et al. reported one or more complications in 58% of procedures, 10% of which were severe [8, 9]. It should be noted that risk of complication was higher with palpable nodes and/or higher patho-logical stage. Nevertheless, some have advocated for early LND in cN0 disease. One retrospective study found 35% 3-year survival in patients who underwent delayed inguinal LND after a period of surveillance versus 84% in patients who underwent early resection [10]. Clinicians must judiciously weigh the risks of pro-cedure morbidity and benefits of survival outcomes in determining management approach.

According to current National Comprehensive Cancer Network (NCCN) guide-lines, the management of non-palpable inguinal nodes is based primarily on the stage of the primary tumor [11]. Low-risk patients (Tis-T1a) can undergo surveil-lance or dynamic sentinel lymph node biopsy (DSNB), while intermediate and high-risk patients ($\geq$T1b) should undergo abdominal/pelvic/chest imaging followed by either ILND or DSNB. This recommendation is based on a study by Slaton et al., which found that pathological tumor stage ($\geq$pT2), vascular invasion, and >50% poorly differentiated cancer were independent risk factors for nodal metastasis [12]. All patients should continue to be surveilled with clinical examination and/or imag-ing on a schedule determined by pathological nodal stage (Table 7.1).

The European Association of Urology (EAU) also risk-stratifies for occult meta-static nodal disease based on stage, histopathological grade, and presence/absence of lymphovascular invasion in the primary tumor [1]. pTa, pTis, and pT1G1 tumors are classified as low-risk, pT1G2 as intermediate risk, and pT1G3 and above as high risk for lymphatic metastasis. Surveillance is recommended only for patients with

Table 7.1 NCCN guidelines for the management of non-palpable inguinal LN

Risk Based on Primary Lesion	Imaging	Treatment		Lymph Node Stage	Surveillance
Low Risk (Tis, Ta, T1a)		Surveillance or DSNB		Nx	Clinical Exam • Years 1-2: every 3 months • Years 3-5: every 6 months
				N0, N1	Clinical Exam • Years 1-2: every 6 months • Years 3-5: every 12 months
				N2, N3	Clinical Exam • Years 1-2: every 3 months • Years 3-5: every 6 months
Intermediate Risk (T1b) or High Risk (>T2)	Abdominal/pelvic (CT or MRI) Chest (X-ray or CT)	ILND or DSNB			Imaging Chest (CT or X-ray) • Years 1-2: every 6 months Abdominal/Pelvic (CT or MRI) • Year 1: every 3 months • Year 2: every 6 months

pTa/Tis disease and certain patients with pT1G1 tumors. Patients with pT1G2 disease or higher should undergo invasive nodal staging, either by DSNB or ILND.

Means of Nodal Staging

The extent of involvement of the inguinal lymph nodes is the most powerful predictor in assessing long-term survival and, therefore, understanding this extent is critical when caring for patients with penile cancer [11]. While inguinal nodes may be non-palpable upon presentation, nomograms and prognostic factors exist that can aid in nodal staging so as to assess the best course of management: surveillance versus inguinal and/or pelvic lymph node dissection (I/P LND). Several of these prognostic factors are listed in Table 7.2.

Regarding tumor grade, it is reported that the risk of inguinal lymph node involvement increases with increased grading: 0–48% for G1 tumors, 32–79% for G2, and 47–100% for G3 [2, 6, 13]. Elsewhere in the literature, similar trends prevail, showing that the tumor grade assists in risk stratification of inguinal lymph node involvement [14, 15].

Additionally, the histology of the primary tumor may also be a predictor of inguinal lymph node involvement. Histologies such as basaloid, sarcomatoid, adenosquamous, and poorly differentiated types have been found to have a higher

Table 7.2 Prognostic factors for predicting presence of regional lymph node involvement

Prognostic factor	Summary	Further reading
Tumor grade	Risk of inguinal lymph node involvement increases with higher grades	Ficarra et al. (2010); Unadkat et al. (2021); Kamel et al. (2019); Graafland et al. (2010); Solsona et al. (2021)
Tumor histology	Histologies such as basaloid, sarcomatoid, adenosquamous, and poorly differentiated types have been found to have a higher incidence of inguinal lymph node involvement	Kamel et al. (2019); Clark et al. (2014)
Lymphovascular invasion	Presence of lymphovascular invasion increases the risk of regional lymph node involvement	Clark et al. (2014); Kamel et al. (2019); Unadkat et al. (2021)
Lymphatic and vascular embolization of tumor	Presence of lymphatic or vascular embolization increases the risk of regional lymph node involvement.	Ficarra et al. (2010); Zhu et al. (2007)
Biomarkers such as p53, cadherin, metalloproteinase-9, squamous cell carcinoma antigen, and Ki-67	Biomarkers may be predictive of inguinal lymph node involvement; however, more research is necessary.	James and Wright (2021); Zhu et al. (2007)

incidence of pN+ while histologies such as verrucous, warty, and papillary were found to have the lowest incidence [13] (Clark et al. 2014).

Lymphovascular invasion and lymphatic and/or vascular embolization have also been found to be strong predictors of regional node involvement [2, 6, 11, 13, 16]. In patients with high- and intermediate-risk disease with lymphovascular invasion, regional lymph node involvement ranged from 68–73% [11]. For patients with lymphatic or venous embolization, Ficarra et al. found that 62–83.3% and 69–89%, respectively, had lymph node metastases [2]. For patients without lymphatic or venous embolization, 17–30.6% and 24–43.8%, respectively, had lymph node metastases [2].

Biomarkers such as those listed in Table 7.2 may also be predictive of lymph node involvement; more research is required into these prognostic factors [16, 17]. Serum biomarkers have shown promising results and are expected to become part of risk stratification of many malignancies, including penile cancer, in the future.

As a means of utilizing some of the prognostic factors discussed above, nomograms have been created to predict presence of regional lymph node involvement [2, 13, 18, 19]. For example, the nomogram developed by Ficarra et al. in 2006 combined variables such as clinical stage, tumor thickness, and histologic grade [19]. However, Kamel et al. have argued that this nomogram is not externally validated. Elsewhere in the literature, one of the nomograms presented by Kattan et al. combined eight variables: clinical inguinal lymph node stage, pathologic tumor thickness, growth pattern, histologic grade, lymphatic and/or venous embolization, corpora cavernosa infiltration, corpus spongiosum, and/or urethral infiltration [18]. In 2010, Ficarra et al. argued that a nomogram such as this may improve accuracy of prediction of nodal disease [2].

Aside from prognostic factors and nomograms, the use of imaging and biopsy in determining regional node involvement is widely debated in the literature [6, 11, 13, 20, 21]. Notably, although there have been improvements in contemporary imaging in past years, imaging modalities such as CT or MRI have been shown to be unreliable in patients with non-palpable lymph nodes [6, 11, 20]. Instead of imaging, for patients with non-palpable lymph nodes, some studies have recommended the use of dynamic sentinel lymph node biopsy (DSNB) [13, 21]. However, due to its technical complexity, this procedure should be reserved for use at high-volume, tertiary care centers [21].

Dynamic Sentinel Lymph Node Biopsy (DSNB)

In order to potentially decrease the complications due to surgical staging, the dynamic sentinel lymph node biopsy (DSNB) has been presented as a less invasive, less morbid procedure to assess lymph node involvement and detect potential metastasis in patients without known inguinal lymph node involvement [22, 23].

This procedure identifies and resects the sentinel lymph node, which is "the first lymph node on a direct drainage pathway from the primary tumor" [23]. A concept first introduced by urologist Ramon Cabanas in 1977, the procedure was first performed by Horenblas et al. in penile cancer patients by using a radioactive colloid and patent blue dye in 1994 [22–24]. Initially, a biopsy was performed on the lymph node medial to the superficial epigastric vein and superomedial to the junction of the saphenous and femoral vein, which was defined as *the* sentinel lymph node for penile cancer. Negative pathology in this sentinel node was considered to preclude metastasis to other nodes. Unfortunately, this procedure did not account for the anatomic variability in patients, and false negative rates of up to 50% were reported [25, 26]. Over time, DSNB was introduced; the "dynamic" aspect signifies the use of lymphoscintigraphy and intradermal blue dye injections to more accurately identify the sentinel lymph node in individual patients. However, initial studies continued to report elevated false negative rates of 17–22% [24]. Major modifications to DSNB have been established since, including: the use of fine needle aspiration cytology prior to DSNB, expanded histopathological analysis, surgical exploration of nonvisualized nodes, and intraoperative palpation of the wound [27]. Since these advances, false negative rates have dropped down to as low as 4.6% [28–30]. Both the NCCN and EAU now recommend DSNB for patients with intermediate-high risk primary tumors and clinically non-palpable lymph nodes.

DSNB procedures have become relatively standardized across high-volume centers [31]. The patient receives a 99 m-Technetium-nanocolloid tracer in combination with vital blue dye, then undergoes dynamic lymphoscintigraphy (after 10–20, and 120 minutes) and single-photon emission computed tomography/CT (after 120 minutes). The sentinel node(s) identified by either/both modalities are biopsied. A gamma ray probe is also used intraoperatively for enhanced detection of nodes. When performed by experienced clinicians, the unilateral nonvisualization rates range from 12–19%, but bilateral nonvisualization rates are low at 0–2% [23]. In a study by Sahdev et al., repeat DSNB at a later date in patients with nonvisualized nodes was successful in 6/7 cases (86%) [32]. The authors thus recommend repeat DSNB in nonvisualized patients with the option of close clinical and imaging surveillance in patients with low-risk disease (<pT1 G3). In the case of nonvisualization on repeat DSNB, patients should proceed with ILND. Omorphos et al. also demonstrated that DSNB can be performed as a delayed procedure after the primary tumor has been removed (mean of 85.9 days) with comparable nonvisualization and false negative rates to DSNB at time of penile surgery [33].

Morbidity from DSNB including infection, lymphocele/seroma formation, and lymphedema is often less severe. Morbidity rates are significantly lower at 5.7–21%, with the majority representing minor complications compared to that of ILND. Future advances in DNSB being studied include the use of fluorescent indocyanine green dye and near-infrared imaging, as well as the use of super-paramagnetic iron oxide nanoparticles in replacement of radioactive tracers [34–36].

Surgical Approaches

ILND is an essential step in caring for patients with intermediate to high-risk primary tumors. Traditionally, the surgery has been done via open approach with an incision 2 cm below the inguinal ligament. The anatomical landmarks for standard ILND template are the inguinal ligament superiorly, the adductor longus muscle medially, sartorius muscle laterally, and the apex of the femoral triangle inferiorly (Fig. 7.1). The dissection sometimes involves ligation and excision of the proximal greater saphenous vein and complete dissection of the femoral vessels within the femoral triangle. Sartorius muscle can be mobilized for coverage of the femoral vessels if needed.

The rates of complications are variable among different studies in part due to differences in methodologies and definitions. Additionally, multiple studies have described the use of different modified templated, or utilization of minimally invasive surgical approaches to reduce the associated high morbidity and long convalescence. Videoscopic endoscopic inguinal lymphadenectomy (VEIL) and robotic videoscopic endoscopic inguinal lymphadenectomy (RVEIL) have been utilized to perform ILND in penile cancer patients with non-palpable inguinal lymph nodes. In these techniques, the long surgical incision in the groin crease, which has a high risk

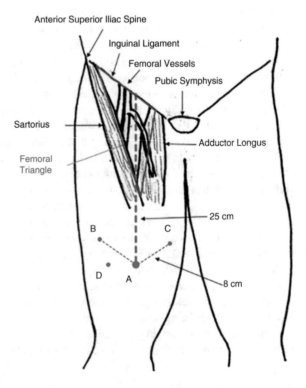

Fig. 7.1 ILND template borders and port sites for minimally invasive approaches

Anterior Superior Iliac Spine

Inguinal Ligament

Femoral Vessels

Pubic Symphysis

Sartorius

Adductor Longus

Femoral Triangle

25 cm

B

C

D   A

8 cm

of dehiscence and infection, is avoided and instead the ports are placed more cau-
dally, and extraction site is smaller and is away from the groin crease (Figs. 7.1
and 7.2).

When comparing VEIL to open ILND, Tobias-Machado and colleagues described
a significant decrease in wound complication (0% vs. 50% $p = 0.02$) as well as a
trend toward less overall complication rates (20% vs. 70% $p = 0.06$) [37], concor-
dant with findings reported by other investigators. Similarly, Singh et al. reported
lower complication rates with RVEIL compared to open ILND (2% vs. 17%,
$p < 0.05$) [38].

Minimally invasive technologies seem to result in faster recovery and less complication rate; factors that can make the surgery more appealing for both the
patients and providers. But how do these approaches compare when oncologic
outcomes are considered? Nodal yield is routinely used as a surrogate for ILND's
oncological adequacy. Multiple single-institutional case-control series have evaluated the oncological adequacy of VEIL and RVEIL, using retrieved nodal count
and inguinal recurrence as measures for oncologic quality. These studies appear to
suggest that minimally invasive techniques can lead to similar oncologic outcomes
when compared to open technique. Another benefit of minimally invasive techniques is that physicians can deliver more timely adjuvant therapies in patients at
high risk of relapse due to lower risk of wound healing complications and shorter
recovery time.

Fig. 7.2 Postoperative
wounds and nodal yield
after VEIL approach
to ILND

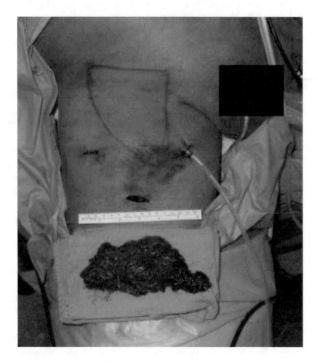

References

1. Hakenberg O, Compérat E, Minhas S, et al. EAU guidelines on penile cancer. Presented at the EAU Guidelines. Edn. presented at the EAU Annual Congress Barcelona, 2019.
2. Ficarra V, Akduman B, Bouchot O, et al. Prognostic factors in penile cancer. Urology. 2010;76:S66.
3. Yang J, Pan Z, He Y, et al. Competing-risks model for predicting the prognosis of penile cancer based on the SEER database. Cancer Med. 2019;8:7881.
4. O'Brien JS, Perera M, Manning T, et al. Penile cancer: contemporary lymph node management. J Urol. 2017;197:1387.
5. Horenblas S, van Tinteren H, Delemarre JF, et al. Squamous cell carcinoma of the penis: accuracy of tumor, nodes and metastasis classification system, and role of lymphangiography, computerized tomography scan and fine needle aspiration cytology. J Urol. 1991;146:1279.
6. Unadkat P, Fleishman A, Olumi AF, et al. Contemporary incidence and predictors of occult inguinal lymph node metastases in men with Clinically Node-Negative (cN0) Penile Cancer. Urology. 2021;153:221–7.
7. Spiess PE, Hernandez MS, Pettaway CA. Contemporary inguinal lymph node dissection: minimizing complications. World J Urol. 2009;27:205.
8. Gopman JM, Djajadiningrat RS, Baumgarten AS, et al. Predicting postoperative complications of inguinal lymph node dissection for penile cancer in an international multicentre cohort. BJU Int. 2015;116:196.
9. Stuiver MM, Djajadiningrat RS, Graafland NM, et al. Early wound complications after inguinal lymphadenectomy in penile cancer: a historical cohort study and risk-factor analysis. Eur Urol. 2013;64:486.
10. Kroon B, Horenblas S, Lont A, et al. Patients with penile carcinoma benefit from immediate resection of clinically occult lymph node metastases. J Urol. 2005;173:816.
11. Flaig TW. NCCN Guidelines Version 2. 2020 Penile Cancer. NCCN, 2020.
12. Slaton JW, Morgenstern N, Levy DA, et al. Tumor stage, vascular invasion and the percentage of poorly differentiated cancer: independent prognosticators for inguinal lymph node metastasis in penile squamous cancer. J Urol. 2001;165(4):1138–42.
13. Kamel MH, Khalil MI, Davis R, et al. Management of the clinically negative (cN0) groin penile cancer patient: a review. Urology. 2019;131:5.
14. Graafland NM, Lam W, Leijte JA, et al. Prognostic factors for occult inguinal lymph node involvement in penile carcinoma and assessment of the high-risk EAU subgroup: a two-institution analysis of 342 clinically node-negative patients. Eur Urol. 2010;58:742.
15. Solsona E, Iborra I, Rubio J, et al. Prospective validation of the association of local tumor stage and grade as a predictive factor for occult lymph node micrometastasis in patients with penile carcinoma and clinically negative inguinal lymph nodes. J Urol. 2001;165:1506.
16. Zhu Y, Zhou XY, Yao XD, et al. The prognostic significance of p53, Ki-67, epithelial cadherin and matrix metalloproteinase-9 in penile squamous cell carcinoma treated with surgery. BJU Int. 2007;100:204.
17. James AC, Wright JL. What is next for penile carcinoma? Presented at the Urologic Oncology-Seminars And Original Investigations, 2021.
18. Kattan MW, Ficarra V, Artibani W, et al. Nomogram predictive of cancer specific survival in patients undergoing partial or total amputation for squamous cell carcinoma of the penis. J Urol. 2006;175:2103.
19. Ficarra V, Zattoni F, Artibani W, et al. Nomogram predictive of pathological inguinal lymph node involvement in patients with squamous cell carcinoma of the penis. J Urol. 2006;175:1700.
20. Heyns CF, Fleshner N, Sangar V, et al. Management of the lymph nodes in penile cancer. Urology. 2010;76:S43.
21. Nabavizadeh R, Petrinec B, Necchi A, et al. Utility of minimally invasive technology for inguinal lymph node dissection in penile cancer. J Clin Med. 2020;9:2501.

22. Perdonà S, Autorino R, De Sio M, et al. Dynamic sentinel node biopsy in clinically node-negative penile cancer versus radical inguinal lymphadenectomy: a comparative study. Urology. 2005;66:1282.
23. Wever L, de Vries H-M, van der Poel H, et al. Minimally invasive evaluation of the clinically negative inguinal node in penile cancer: dynamic sentinel node biopsy. Presented at the Urologic Oncology: Seminars and Original Investigations, 2020.
24. Zou Z-J, Liu Z-H, Tang L-Y, et al. Radiocolloid-based dynamic sentinel lymph node biopsy in penile cancer with clinically negative inguinal lymph node: an updated systematic review and meta-analysis. Int Urol Nephrol. 2016;48:2001.
25. Pettaway CA, Pisters LL, Dinney CP, et al. Sentinel lymph node dissection for penile carcinoma: the MD Anderson Cancer Center experience. J Urol. 1995;154:1999.
26. Mcdougal WS, Kirchner FK Jr, Edwards RH, et al. Treatment of carcinoma of the penis: the case for primary lymphadenectomy. J Urol. 1986;136:38.
27. Kroon B, Horenblas S, Estourgie S, et al. How to avoid false-negative dynamic sentinel node procedures in penile carcinoma. J Urol. 2004;171:2191.
28. Jakobsen JK, Krarup KP, Sommer P, et al. DaPeCa-1: diagnostic accuracy of sentinel lymph node biopsy in 222 patients with penile cancer at four tertiary referral centres–a national study from Denmark. BJU Int. 2016;117:235.
29. Lam W, Alnajjar HM, La-Touche S, et al. Dynamic sentinel lymph node biopsy in patients with invasive squamous cell carcinoma of the penis: a prospective study of the long-term outcome of 500 inguinal basins assessed at a single institution. Eur Urol. 2013;63:657.
30. Leijte JA, Kroon BK, Olmos RAV, et al. Reliability and safety of current dynamic sentinel node biopsy for penile carcinoma. Eur Urol. 2007;52:170.
31. Thomas A, Necchi A, Muneer A, et al. Penile cancer. Nat Rev Dis Primers. 2021;7:1.
32. Sahdev V, Albersen M, Christodoulidou M, et al. Management of non-visualization following dynamic sentinel lymph node biopsy for squamous cell carcinoma of the penis. BJU Int. 2017;119:573.
33. Omorphos S, Saad Z, Arya M, et al. Feasibility of performing dynamic sentinel lymph node biopsy as a delayed procedure in penile cancer. World J Urol. 2016;34:329.
34. Brouwer OR, van den Berg NS, Mathéron HM, et al. A hybrid radioactive and fluorescent tracer for sentinel node biopsy in penile carcinoma as a potential replacement for blue dye. Eur Urol. 2014;65:600.
35. Winter A, Woenkhaus J, Wawroschek F. A novel method for intraoperative sentinel lymph node detection in prostate cancer patients using superparamagnetic iron oxide nanoparticles and a handheld magnetometer: the initial clinical experience. Ann Surg Oncol. 2014;21:4390.
36. Douek M, Klaase J, Monypenny I, et al. Sentinel node biopsy using a magnetic tracer versus standard technique: the SentiMAG Multicentre Trial. Ann Surg Oncol. 2014;21:1237.
37. Tobias-Machado M, Tavares A, Ornellas AA, Molina WR, Juliano RV, Wroclawski ER. Video endoscopic inguinal lymphadenectomy: a new minimally invasive procedure for radical management of inguinal nodes in patients with penile squamous cell carcinoma. J Urol. 2007;177:953–8.
38. Singh A, Jaipuria J, Goel A, Shah S, Bhardwaj R, Baidya S, Jain J, Jain C, Rawal S. Comparing outcomes of robotic and open inguinal lymph node dissection in patients with carcinoma of the penis. J Urol. 2018;199:1518–25.

Chapter 8
Management of Bulky Inguinal/Pelvic Metastases in Squamous Penile Cancer

Mohamed E. Ahmed, Vidhu B. Joshi, Curtis A. Pettaway, R. Jeffrey Karnes, and Philippe E. Spiess

Introduction

In 2017, the American Joint Committee on Cancer (AJCC) released a revised *AJCC Cancer Staging Manual* (8th edition) that included updates to the TNM classification for penile squamous cell carcinoma (PSCC) with respect to nodal disease [1, 2]. Specifically, the AJCC now separates pN1 and pN2 nodal disease based on the number of nodes (≤ 2 for pN1, versus ≥ 3 for pN2) and laterality (unilateral nodes for pN1, versus any number of bilateral nodes for pN2). Patients that demonstrate extranodal extension (ENE) or pelvic lymph node metastases are classified as pN3. These changes underscore the large differences in outcomes for patients with unilateral versus bilateral nodal disease, with 5-year overall survival (OS) rates of ~80% compared to 10–20% among patients with unilateral inguinal versus bilateral inguinal or pelvic nodal disease, respectively [3]. In this chapter, we will discuss the management of clinical N2-N3 PSCC that equates to penile cancer in the setting of bulky inguinal or pelvic lymph node metastases.

Mohamed E. Ahmed and Vidhu B. Joshi contributed equally with all other contributors.

M. E. Ahmed · V. B. Joshi · R. J. Karnes
Department of Urology, Mayo Clinic, Rochester, MN, USA
e-mail: Mohamed.Ahmed@mayo.edu; Joshi.Vidhu@mayo.edu; Karnes.R@mayo.edu

C. A. Pettaway
Department of Urology, The University of Texas MD Anderson Cancer Center, Houston, TX, USA
e-mail: cpettawa@mdanderson.org

P. E. Spiess (✉)
Department of Genito-Urinary Oncology, Department of Tumor Biology, H. Lee Moffitt Cancer Center and Research Institute, Tampa, FL, USA
e-mail: Philippe.Spiess@moffitt.org

© The Author(s), under exclusive license to Springer Nature Switzerland AG 2021
P. E. Spiess, A. Necchi (eds.), *Penile Carcinoma*,
https://doi.org/10.1007/978-3-030-82060-2_8

Advances in Diagnosis

Given that the number, laterality, and location of lymph node metastases are prognostic predictors of PSCC, rapid and meticulous evaluation of palpable lymph nodes plays a critical role in properly managing locally advanced penile cancer [4–6]. Thus, an ultrasound/CT-guided biopsy or fine needle aspiration (FNA) is usually performed to confirm metastatic disease in patients with palpable or radiographically suspicious inguinal lymphadenopathy [7].

Additionally, major recent advances have been made in noninvasive techniques for evaluating suspicious nodes and assessing the extent of lymph node involvement. A meta-analysis looking at the accuracy of 18F-FDG PET/CT in detecting inguinal lymph node metastases among patients with clinically suspicious inguinal lymphadenopathy revealed pooled sensitivity and specificity rates of 96% and 92%, respectively [8]. Additionally, among patients who have biopsy-proven lymph node involvement, comprehensive evaluation is required to determine the spread of nodal disease, including laterality, possible extranodal extension, and pelvic lymph node involvement [9, 10]. In a single center study, Lughezzani et al. investigated predictors of pelvic lymph node involvement in 142 penile cancer patients with 188 positive inguinal lymph nodes [11]. The authors reported that the number of inguinal lymph nodes ($\geq$3 nodes), the diameter of the inguinal lymph node ($\geq$30 mm), and extranodal involvement are significant predictors of pelvic lymph node involvement [11]. In addition, in a multicenter study, Zargar-Shoshtari et al. studied predictors of bilateral pelvic lymph node dissection in penile cancer patients with confirmed inguinal lymph node metastases [12]. In univariate and multivariate logistic regression analyses, the authors noted that detection of $\geq$4 positive inguinal lymph node metastases was the only significant predictor of bilateral lymph node metastases [12].

As will be discussed later in this chapter, these features help determine the treatment approach.

Surgical Management

Following a positive ultrasound/CT-guided percutaneous biopsy of palpable lymph node(s) in the setting of bulky inguinal/pelvic nodal metastases(i.e., unilateral adenopathy$\geq$4 cm, fixed or bilateral nodes), the National Comprehensive Cancer Network (NCCN) recommends multimodal therapy in the form of neoadjuvant chemotherapy (discussed later) followed by lymph node dissection (LND) for patients with surgically resectable disease [10]. If a biopsy yields a negative result (usually in the setting of unilateral adenopathy with node size<4 cm), an excisional biopsy is recommended by the NCCN to confirm the negative finding. In this section, we will briefly summarize the NCCN guidelines on the surgical treatment of biopsy confirmed N2-N3 disease, as well as review the literature on oncologic outcomes and postoperative complications. In this chapter, all NCCN guidelines are category 2A (unless otherwise indicated), meaning the guidelines are based on low-level evidence and there is consensus within the NCCN regarding its use.

Surgical Approach

Inguinal lymph node dissection (ILND) and pelvic lymph node dissection (PLND) are the standard modalities (+/− chemotherapy or radiotherapy) for the management of locally advanced penile cancer to achieve locoregional control of the disease.

Inguinal Lymph Node Dissection There are several approaches to ILND among patients with clinically evident disease with various incisions utilized.

Full-template ILND. We commonly recommend a horizontal incision below the level of the inguinal ligament. The boundaries of the standard full-template ILND are shown in Fig. 8.1 and is 2–3 cm above the inguinal ligament; superiorly, the apex of the femoral triangle; inferiorly, the midpoint of the adductor longus muscle (about a 15 cm line extending from the pubic tubercle); medially, and the midpoint

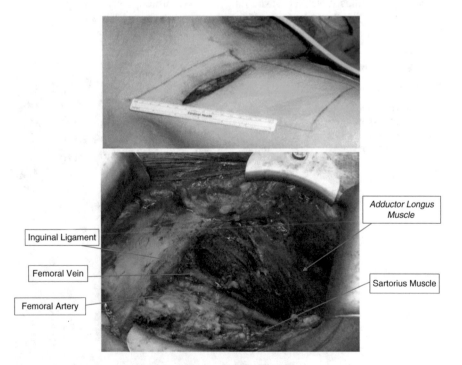

Fig. 8.1 Markings and boundaries of inguinal lymph node dissection in penile cancer

of the sartorius muscle (about a 20 cm line extending from anterior superior iliac spine); laterally [13]. The sartorius muscle can be transposed to cover the femoral vessels if there is a concern that the overlying skin may not be viable on the long term or after adjuvant therapy (Fig. 8.2a). In the setting where the overlying skin is involved or fixed to an underlying inguinal mass, a myocutaneous flap (Fig. 8.2b) can be used to cover large skin defects where overlying skin is resected. Among patients with lower volume palpable inguinal metastases (i.e., nodes <4 cm, cN2 or less), a therapeutic open fascial-sparing, saphenous-sparing approach has also been reported with longer-term follow-up [14]. This dissection spares the fascia lata of the thigh and preserves the saphenous vein, but it also obviates the need for intraoperative frozen sections because it removes the deep nodes within the fossa ovalis around the femoral vessels. In one study evaluating this approach, 104 patients underwent 201 inguinal dissections for cN0-cN2 (minimal disease). At a median follow-up of 36 months, only a single inguinal recurrence was noted [14].

Pelvic Lymph Node Dissection There is a lack of consensus on the boundaries and the extent of pelvic lymph node dissection in patients with penile cancer, and this is due in big part to the lack of sufficient mapping studies of the location and extent of penile cancer pelvic lymph node metastases [15]. The currently used approach to PLND usually includes the removal of the distal common iliac lymph nodes, external iliac lymph nodes, and obturator lymph nodes [10, 15, 16].

Multiple studies have demonstrated that LND prolongs survival, particularly when a complete dissection is performed removing the nodes within specified

Fig. 8.2 (a) Sartorius muscle flap pulled over the vessels following deep inguinal lymph node dissection, (b) showing anterolateral thigh myocutaneous flap in place

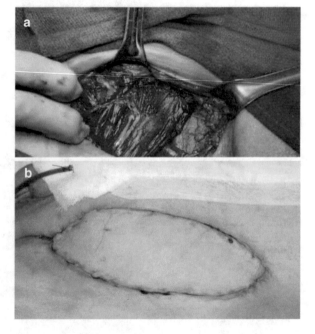

boundaries [11, 12, 17–22]. This type of dissection is usually reflected in a higher node count. For example, a retrospective analysis by Li et al. demonstrated that the removal of ≥16 lymph nodes was an independent predictor of disease-specific survival (DSS) on multivariate analysis [17]. Similarly, an analysis of the National Cancer Database showed that the removal of >15 lymph nodes was associated with greater OS[19]. In addition to the number of lymph nodes removed, studies have demonstrated improved outcomes in patients that undergo bilateral LND for unilateral inguinal nodal disease with high-risk features like ENE or pelvic nodes. For example, an international, multi-center retrospective analysis showed improved OS among patients with unilateral inguinal and pelvic metastases who underwent bilateral PLND, versus those who only underwent ipsilateral PLND [20]. Based on these findings, the NCCN recommends a bilateral PLND for patients with ≥4 positive inguinal lymph nodes [10].

The most recent NCCN guidelines for the management of palpable, bulky inguinal lymph nodes and pelvic lymph nodes are summarized in Table 8.1 [10]. In general, following neoadjuvant chemotherapy, ILND in the setting of both unilateral and bilateral inguinal metastases is recommended. These patients should be offered upfront ILND if they are ineligible for neoadjuvant chemotherapy. In the setting of nodal metastases limited to the inguinal region, the NCCN guidelines also recommends expanding the surgical management of these patients to include a PLND, especially in patients who exhibit ≥4 cm unilateral inguinal lymph nodes, those that are <4 cm and fixed, or bilateral lymph nodes. PLND can be done concomitantly with ILND based on intraoperative findings (further details in Table 8.1), or during a second procedure following ILND. Notably, for patients with ≥4 cm unilateral

Table 8.1 Summary of NCCN guidelines on the surgical management of biopsy-proven bulky inguinal and pelvic lymph node metastases following neoadjuvant chemotherapy

	ILND	PLND
Mobile unilateral inguinal lymph nodes ≥ 4 cm	Recommended [a]	Consider unilateral if ≥2 ipsilateral positive inguinal nodes or presence of ENE
Fixed unilateral inguinal lymph nodes OR, Fixed/mobile bilateral inguinal lymph nodes < 4 cm	Recommended [b]	Recommended [b] Note: Consider bilateral if ≥4 positive inguinal nodes (ipsilaterally and contralaterally, combined)
Pelvic lymph nodes	For these patients, consolidation surgery in the form of bilateral ILND combined with unilateral or bilateral PLND is recommended [c]	

Abbreviations: *ILND* inguinal lymph node dissection, *NCCN* National Comprehensive Cancer Network, *PLND* pelvic lymph node dissection

[a] ILND recommended with or without prior induction chemotherapy

[b] Neoadjuvant chemotherapy preferred with subsequent ILND/PLND performed in response to therapy. ILND should be considered upfront among patients that are not eligible for chemotherapy, if otherwise resectable

[c] Recommended only for neoadjuvant chemotherapy responders

inguinal lymph nodes, or those that are <4 cm and fixed, or bilateral lymph nodes, surgery is only recommended for those who responded to neoadjuvant chemotherapy or were ineligible for neoadjuvant chemotherapy at presentation. Similarly, patients who have biopsy-proven pelvic metastases and are surgical candidates, neoadjuvant chemotherapy is given upfront (discussed later) followed by bilateral ILND combined with either unilateral or bilateral PLND (Table 8.1) [10].

With respect to postoperative complications, ILND and PLND have historically been associated with high complication rates between 42–57% [23]. It has been suggested that approximately 50% of patients will experience a postoperative complication, with the most common complications including wound infection, wound dehiscence, wound necrosis, lymphocele, lymphoedema, hematoma, and venous thromboembolism [23]. Differences in complication rates can be attributed to several factors including the approach used (i.e., open versus minimally invasive), extent of dissection (i.e., unilateral versus bilateral, +/– pelvic), the purpose of the LND (i.e., prophylactic versus therapeutic), and differences in perioperative care. While prospective and randomized trials are warranted to evaluate the impact of these differences on postoperative outcomes, the overall complication rate for LND for PSCC is declining [23].

Neoadjuvant Chemotherapy

As mentioned previously, neoadjuvant chemotherapy prior to ILND/PLND is recommended by the NCCN for those who are eligible, as surgery alone is unlikely to be curative [24]. Specifically, four cycles of TIP (paclitaxel, ifosfamide, and cisplatin) is the preferred regimen [10]. This recommendation is based on findings from the phase II clinical trial by Pagliaro et al. on neoadjuvant chemotherapy for PSCC. This single-arm, non-randomized, prospective phase II trial of the TIP regimen was performed at a single institution in 30 patients with cN2/N3 PSCC [25]. The key findings from this landmark trial included an objective response rate (ORR) of 50%, pathological complete response (pCR) in 10% of patients, and 30% of patients remaining free of recurrence at a median follow-up of 34 months. This trial provided support for the efficacy of multimodal management of locally advanced PSCC, given that response to neoadjuvant chemotherapy was significantly associated with improved OS (median 17.1 months) and time to progression (TTP) (median 8.1 months), as well as the absence of bilateral residual tumor and ENE – both of which are described as predictors of poor prognosis. Thus, these findings are consistent with other studies that suggest neoadjuvant chemotherapy also has prognostic value [26–28]. Of note, the TIP regimen was well-tolerated with grade 3 infections being the most common adverse event. Postsurgical complication rates were also comparable to historical data on ILND, providing further support for the feasibility of a multimodal approach to locally advanced penile cancer. Despite being the only prospective study published to date, the findings reported by Pagliaro et al. are consistent with those described in a recent systematic review of retrospective studies on neoadjuvant chemotherapy. Specifically, the pooled analysis demonstrated an objective response rate of 53% for taxane-based chemotherapy regimens, of which the majority included cisplatin [29].

In order to further elucidate the value of neoadjuvant chemotherapy in a randomized trial, the International Penile Advanced Cancer Trial (InPACT) was launched internationally in 2017 to accrue 400 patients over a 5-year period, with recent accrual goals adjusted to 200 patients to achieve similar study endpoints. In this study, patients with cTany/cN1–3/M0 PSCC will be randomized into one of three arms: (1) ILND alone, (2) neoadjuvant chemotherapy followed by ILND, or (3) neoadjuvant chemoradiation followed by ILND. The primary outcome measure is overall survival, and the major secondary outcome measures include disease-specific survival, toxicity, disease-free survival, surgical complications, and overall quality of life (QOL) [30].

Adjuvant Chemotherapy

Per NCCN guidelines, adjuvant chemotherapy is only recommended as an option in patients with mobile unilateral inguinal lymph nodes ≥4 cm who demonstrated ≥2 positive nodes or ENE at the time of ILND and did not receive neoadjuvant chemotherapy (i.e., pN2-N3). In this setting, either the TIP regimen or 5-fluorouracil plus cisplatin can be administered. This recommendation is based on limited retrospective studies of adjuvant chemotherapy in patients with pelvic lymph metastases [31–33]. Specifically, a recent multicenter retrospective study reported a significant improvement in OS exclusively among patients with pN3 disease due to positive pelvic lymph nodes [32]. Similarly, another multicenter retrospective study demonstrated an improved median OS of 21.7 months versus 10.1 months in patients who received adjuvant therapy versus those that did not, respectively [33]. Thus, there is some data to support the use of adjuvant chemotherapy among patients with pN2-N3 penile cancer, and this is supported by both the NCCN and the European Association of Urology (EAU) penile cancer guidelines [34].

Radiotherapy and Chemoradiotherapy

With respect to the use of radiotherapy in the management of bulky inguinal and pelvic nodal PSCC, the NCCN recommends radiotherapy or chemoradiotherapy as an option among patients with surgically unresectable disease as well as a consideration among patients that are not eligible for combination chemotherapy [10]. Adjuvant radiotherapy can also be offered as an option to patients following ILND and PLND, although the literature is sparse and there is a lack of consensus. For example, a 2018 study of the National Cancer Database demonstrated an improvement in OS following adjuvant therapy post-ILND [35]. Similarly, another retrospective study showed a significant difference in disease-specific survival among patients who received adjuvant radiation to the pelvis (14.4 months) versus those who did not receive adjuvant pelvic radiation (8 months) [36]. In contrast, a systematic review of studies on adjuvant radiation did not find any significant improvement in recurrence or survival among the 1606 men across the selected retrospective studies [37]. Thus, further prospective studies are warranted to examine the utility of radiotherapy and chemoradiotherapy for locally advanced penile cancer.

Of note, the second randomization in the previously discussed InPACT trial (specifically called InPACT Pelvis) involves assigning patients at high risk of pelvic involvement at the time of ILND to one of four arms: (1) adjuvant chemoradiation with PLND in radiation-naive patients, (2) adjuvant chemoradiation to the pelvis without PLND in prior radiation-naïve patients, (3) PLND alone in patients who already received neoadjuvant chemoradiation, or (4) surveillance alone in patients who received neoadjuvant chemoradiation. The findings from this portion of the InPACT trial will provide further data on the efficacy of chemoradiation and whether or not PLND provides any additional benefit in terms of cancer control [30].

Investigational Treatment Modalities

Due to the poor prognosis associated with locally advanced PSCC involving bulky nodal metastases and a limited number of treatment options that lack higher-level evidence based on prospective studies, efforts have been made to explore other treatment modalities. For example, Necchi et al. studied the use of dacomitinib, an epidermal growth factor receptor (EGFR) tyrosine kinase inhibitor (TKI), in a phase II single-arm study of 28 chemo-naive patients with cN2-N3 or M1 disease – of these, 71% had inguinal or lymph node metastases only. Among all patients, the study reported an ORR of 32% and a 12-month OS rate of 55%. Within the locally advanced PSCC patients, a progression-free survival (PFS) rate and 12-month OS rate of 36% and 64% was observed, respectively [38]. While dacomitinib was well-tolerated in this cohort, the ORR observed in patients with locally advanced PSCC was less than the 50% ORR reported by Pagliaro et al. for the TIP neoadjuvant chemotherapy regimen [25]. Thus, while modest in efficacy, TKI therapy with agents like dacomitinib could be further investigated for patients that are ineligible for chemotherapy or combined with chemotherapy to determine if responses are enhanced.

In addition to TKIs, immune checkpoint blockade (ICI) therapy is being investigated as a potential therapy for advanced PSCC. Biomarker studies have demonstrated the expression of programmed death-ligand 1 (PD-L1) in penile cancer, with one study showing 69.2% of tumors with lymph node metastases being PD-L1-positive [39, 40]. Hahn et al. recently showed that one of three patients receiving single agent pembrolizumab with advanced chemotherapy-resistant disease had a durable response and was alive at >38 months post resection of residual disease. The responding patient exhibited microsatellite instability, which is a known prognostic feature for response among patients receiving immune

Table 8.2 Ongoing clinical trials investigating ICI therapy in the setting of bulky inguinal and pelvic lymph node metastases (cN2-N3)

	ICI agent	Combination therapy (if applicable)	Line of therapy
NCT04224740	Pembrolizumab (anti-PD-1)	Cisplatin/carboplatin plus 5-FU	First-line
NCT03774901	Avelumab (anti-PD-L1)	N/A	Maintenance therapy following chemotherapy for surgically unresectable disease
NCT03686332	Atezolizumab (anti-PD-L1)	Radiotherapy	Surgically unresectable disease
NCT042311981	Retifanlimab (anti-PD-1)	N/A	Surgically unresectable disease

Abbreviations: *ICI* immune checkpoint blockade, *PD-1* programmed cell death protein 1, *PD-L1* programmed death-ligand 1, *5-FU* 5-fluorouracil

checkpoint inhibitors [41]. Based on these and other reports, a number of prospective clinical trials are investigating ICI therapy for advanced penile cancer. Table 8.2 lists the ongoing trials (non-basket) in the setting of advanced penile cancer, including cN2-N3 PSCC.

Conclusion

Due to the poor prognosis associated with bulky inguinal and pelvic lymph node PSCC, patients in this setting must be managed in a multidisciplinary fashion. As discussed in this chapter, this often includes surgery, chemotherapy, and possibly radiotherapy. However, the efficacy of each of these therapies as well as the optimal sequencing and combination of these modalities remain to be investigated in prospective, randomized clinical trials such as InPACT. Currently, clinicians utilize the NCCN or EAU guidelines for the treatment of bulky nodal disease, which are based on lower-level evidence. In addition to evaluating existing treatment options in clinical trials, novel therapies such as TKIs and immune checkpoint blockade should be further investigated. Further advances in management will come about with improved understanding of the biological pathways that drive the disease so that new strategies are developed in addition to prognostic and predictive biomarkers of response.

References

1. Amin MB, et al. AJCC Cancer Staging Manual. 8th edition, Springer International Publishing, Birhauser Verlag AG, Switzerland; 2017.
2. Paner GP, et al. Updates in the eighth edition of the tumor-node-metastasis staging classification for urologic cancers. Eur Urol. 2018;73:560–9. https://doi.org/10.1016/j.eururo.2017.12.018.
3. Pagliaro LC, Crook J. Multimodality therapy in penile cancer: when and which treatments? World J Urol. 2009;27:221–5. https://doi.org/10.1007/s00345-008-0310-z.

4. Ficarra V, Akduman B, Bouchot O, Palou J, Tobias-Machado M. Prognostic factors in penile cancer. Urology. 2010;76:S66–73. https://doi.org/10.1016/j.urology.2010.04.008.

5. Horenblas S, van Tinteren H. Squamous cell carcinoma of the penis. IV. Prognostic factors of survival: analysis of tumor, nodes and metastasis classification system. J Urol. 1994;151:1239–43. https://doi.org/10.1016/s0022-5347(17)35221-7.

6. Srinivas V, Morse MJ, Herr HW, Sogani PC, Whitmore WF Jr. Penile cancer: relation of extent of nodal metastasis to survival. J Urol. 1987;137:880–2. https://doi.org/10.1016/s0022-5347(17)44281-9.

7. Johnston MJ, Nigam R. Recent advances in the management of penile cancer. F1000Res. 2019;8. https://doi.org/10.12688/f1000research.18185.1.

8. Sadeghi R, Gholami H, Zakavi SR, Kakhki VR, Horenblas S. Accuracy of 18F-FDG PET/CT for diagnosing inguinal lymph node involvement in penile squamous cell carcinoma: systematic review and meta-analysis of the literature. Clin Nucl Med. 2012;37:436–41. https://doi.org/10.1097/RLU.0b013e318238f6ea.

9. Thomas A, et al. Penile cancer. Nat Rev Dis Primers. 2021;7:11. https://doi.org/10.1038/s41572-021-00246-5.

10. Network, N. C. C. Penile Cancer. 2021. https://www.nccn.org/professionals/physician_gls/pdf/penile.pdf.

11. Lughezzani G, et al. Relationship between lymph node ratio and cancer-specific survival in a contemporary series of patients with penile cancer and lymph node metastases. BJU Int. 2015;116:727–33. https://doi.org/10.1111/bju.12510.

12. Zargar-Shoshtari K, et al. Establishing criteria for bilateral pelvic lymph node dissection in the Management of Penile Cancer: lessons learned from an international multicenter collaboration. J Urol. 2015;194:696–701. https://doi.org/10.1016/j.juro.2015.03.090.

13. Bevan-Thomas R, Slaton JW, Pettaway CA. Contemporary morbidity from lymphadenectomy for penile squamous cell carcinoma: the M.D. Anderson Cancer Center Experience. J Urol. 2002;167:1638–42.

14. Yao K, et al. Fascia lata preservation during inguinal lymphadenectomy for penile cancer: rationale and outcome. Urology. 2013;82:642–7. https://doi.org/10.1016/j.urology.2013.05.021.

15. Yao K, et al. Lymph node mapping in patients with penile cancer undergoing pelvic lymph node dissection. J Urol. 2021;205:145–51. https://doi.org/10.1097/ju.0000000000001322.

16. Pettaway, CA et al. Chapter 37: Tumors of the Penis. Campbell-Walsh Urology 12th Edition, Elsevier Publishing Group; Netherlands, Amsterdam, 2020.

17. Li ZS, et al. Disease-specific survival after radical lymphadenectomy for penile cancer: prediction by lymph node count and density. Urol Oncol. 2014;32:893–900. https://doi.org/10.1016/j.urolonc.2013.11.008.

18. Joshi SS, et al. Treatment trends and outcomes for patients with lymph node-positive cancer of the penis. JAMA Oncol. 2018;4:643–9. https://doi.org/10.1001/jamaoncol.2017.5608.

19. Soodana-Prakash N, et al. Lymph node yield as a predictor of overall survival following inguinal lymphadenectomy for penile cancer. Urol Oncol. 2018;36:471.e419–27. https://doi.org/10.1016/j.urolonc.2018.07.010.

20. Zargar-Shoshtari K, et al. Extent of pelvic lymph node dissection in penile cancer may impact survival. World J Urol. 2016;34:353–9. https://doi.org/10.1007/s00345-015-1593-5.

21. O'Brien JS, et al. Penile cancer: contemporary lymph node management. J Urol. 2017;197:1387–95. https://doi.org/10.1016/j.juro.2017.01.059.

22. Ball MW, et al. Lymph node density predicts recurrence and death after inguinal lymph node dissection for penile cancer. Investig Clin Urol. 2017;58:20–6. https://doi.org/10.4111/icu.2017.58.1.20.

23. Spiess PE, Hernandez MS, Pettaway CA. Contemporary inguinal lymph node dissection: minimizing complications. World J Urol. 2009;27:205–12. https://doi.org/10.1007/s00345-008-0324-6.

24. Tward J. The case for nonsurgical therapy of nonmetastatic penile cancer. Nat Rev Urol. 2018;15:574–84. https://doi.org/10.1038/s41585-018-0040-y.

25. Pagliaro LC, et al. Neoadjuvant paclitaxel, ifosfamide, and cisplatin chemotherapy for metastatic penile cancer: a phase II study. J Clin Oncol. 2010;28:3851–7. https://doi.org/10.1200/JCO.2010.29.5477.
26. Leijte JA, Kerst JM, Bais E, Antonini N, Horenblas S. Neoadjuvant chemotherapy in advanced penile carcinoma. Eur Urol. 2007;52:488–94. https://doi.org/10.1016/j.eururo.2007.02.006.
27. Zou B, et al. Neoadjuvant therapy combined with a BMP regimen for treating penile cancer patients with lymph node metastasis: a retrospective study in China. J Cancer Res Clin Oncol. 2014;140:1733–8. https://doi.org/10.1007/s00432-014-1720-5.
28. Djajadiningrat RS, Bergman AM, van Werkhoven E, Vegt E, Horenblas S. Neoadjuvant taxane-based combination chemotherapy in patients with advanced penile cancer. Clin Genitourin Cancer. 2015;13:44–9. https://doi.org/10.1016/j.clgc.2014.06.005.
29. Azizi M, et al. Systematic review and meta-analysis-is there a benefit in using neoadjuvant systemic chemotherapy for locally advanced penile squamous cell carcinoma? J Urol. 2020;203:1147–55. https://doi.org/10.1097/JU.0000000000000746.
30. Canter DJ, Nicholson S, Watkin N, Hall E, Pettaway C. The International Penile Advanced Cancer Trial (InPACT): rationale and current status. Eur Urol Focus. 2019;5:706–9. https://doi.org/10.1016/j.euf.2019.05.010.
31. Nicolai N, et al. A combination of cisplatin and 5-fluorouracil with a Taxane in patients who underwent lymph node dissection for nodal metastases from squamous cell carcinoma of the penis: treatment outcome and survival analyses in neoadjuvant and adjuvant settings. Clin Genitourin Cancer. 2016;14:323–30. https://doi.org/10.1016/j.clgc.2015.07.009.
32. Necchi A, et al. Nomogram-based prediction of overall survival after regional lymph node dissection and the role of perioperative chemotherapy in penile squamous cell carcinoma: A retrospective multicenter study. Urol Oncol. 2019;37:531.e537–531.e515, https://doi.org/10.1016/j.urolonc.2019.04.003.
33. Sharma P, et al. Adjuvant chemotherapy is associated with improved overall survival in pelvic node-positive penile cancer after lymph node dissection: a multi-institutional study. Urol Oncol. 2015;33(496):e417–23. https://doi.org/10.1016/j.urolonc.2015.05.008.
34. Hakenberg OW, et al. EAU guidelines on penile cancer: 2014 update. Eur Urol. 2015;67:142–50. https://doi.org/10.1016/j.eururo.2014.10.017.
35. Winters BR, et al. Is there a benefit to adjuvant radiation in stage III penile cancer after lymph node dissection? Findings from the National Cancer Database. Urol Oncol. 2018;36:92.e11–6. https://doi.org/10.1016/j.urolonc.2017.11.005.
36. Tang DH, et al. Adjuvant pelvic radiation is associated with improved survival and decreased disease recurrence in pelvic node-positive penile cancer after lymph node dissection: a multi-institutional study. Urol Oncol. 2017;35:605.e617–23. https://doi.org/10.1016/j.urolonc.2017.06.001.
37. Robinson R, et al. Risks and benefits of adjuvant radiotherapy after inguinal lymphadenectomy in node-positive penile cancer: a systematic review by the European Association of Urology Penile Cancer Guidelines Panel. Eur Urol. 2018;74:76–83. https://doi.org/10.1016/j.eururo.2018.04.003.
38. Necchi A, et al. First-line therapy with dacomitinib, an orally available pan-HER tyrosine kinase inhibitor, for locally advanced or metastatic penile squamous cell carcinoma: results of an open-label, single-arm, single-centre, phase 2 study. BJU Int. 2018;121:348–56. https://doi.org/10.1111/bju.14013.
39. Cocks M, et al. Immune-checkpoint status in penile squamous cell carcinoma: a North American cohort. Hum Pathol. 2017;59:55–61. https://doi.org/10.1016/j.humpath.2016.09.003.
40. De Bacco MW, et al. PD-L1 and p16 expression in penile squamous cell carcinoma from an endemic region. Clin Genitourin Cancer. 2020;18:e254–9. https://doi.org/10.1016/j.clgc.2019.10.014.
41. Hahn, A. W. et al. Pembrolizumab for advanced penile cancer: a case series from a phase II basket trial. Invest New Drugs. 2021. https://doi.org/10.1007/s10637-021-01100-x.

Chapter 9
Neoadjuvant and Adjuvant Multimodality Treatments for Patients with Lymph Node Involvement

Marco Bandini, Peter A. S. Johnstone, and Andrea Necchi

Squamous cell carcinoma of the penis (PSC) is a rare disease, though as with any malignant process, specific attention must be paid to three distinct clinical scenarios: local therapy, regional therapy, and distant metastases; only local therapy has been robustly investigated. In this chapter, we discuss the regional disease process and outline where current and future opportunities may lie.

Radiotherapy

There are very few data and no completed prospective trials available on radiotherapy (RT) in PSC. Given squamous histology and shared relationships with HPV and squamous histology, many clinicians extrapolate data and results from vulvar (VuC) or oropharyngeal cancer (OPC) to PSC. This is unwise. Recent genomic analyses

M. Bandini (✉)
Urological Research Institute, Vita-Salute San Raffaele University, Milan, Italy
e-mail: bandini.marco@hsr.it

P. A. S. Johnstone
Departments of Radiation Oncology and Health Outcomes & Behavior, Moffitt Cancer Center, University of South Florida, Tampa, FL, USA
e-mail: Peter.Johnstone@moffitt.org

A. Necchi
Vita-Salute San Raffaele University, IRCCS San Raffaele Hospital and Scientific Institute, Milan, Italy
e-mail: Andrea.Necchi@istitutotumori.mi.it

© The Author(s), under exclusive license to Springer Nature Switzerland AG 2021
P. E. Spiess, A. Necchi (eds.), *Penile Carcinoma*,
https://doi.org/10.1007/978-3-030-82060-2_9

have revealed that both primary PSC lesions [1] and nodal tissue [2] have genomic radiosensitivity signatures far different from HPV-positive OPC. In fact, mean radiosensitivity of PSC is very close to that of melanoma: one of the most resistant tumor subtypes. This may explain the disparate results of the few analyses in the literature [3–6].

Likely because of this, there remain no good data supporting preoperative RT in any case, or postoperative RT for pN1 or pN2 PeCa [7]. Because of this, it is not surprising that analysis of the US National Cancer Database reveals that adjuvant RT is more frequently provided to pN1/pN2 PSC in the community than in academic centers [8]. Simply adding adjuvant RT because we would do so for VuC or OPC is insufficient rationale when the data are analyzed.

Nevertheless, there are some patient populations for which adjuvant nodal basin RT may be of benefit. The first case is if there is extranodal extension of disease (ENE). Graafland and associates described that ENE portends poorer cancer-specific survival in PSC patients [9], but did not comment on the role of RT. In our international, multi-institutional analysis [10], patients without ENE had better relapse-free survival with RT: $p = 0.016$ for groin RT and $p = 0.006$ for inguinopelvic RT. Overall survival was improved by adjuvant inguinopelvic RT ($p = 0.037$). This was not the case for patients with ENE. These patients had no local-regional benefit to adjuvant RT but did experience a disease-specific survival benefit to inguinopelvic RT ($p = 0.041$).

Thus, delivering adjuvant inguinopelvic RT provided a distinct local control benefit only for ENE (−) patients. This is because the disease burden in ENE (+) patients may be too extreme for current RT dosing regimens of 50–54 Gy. In our genomic analysis, we modeled that a standard dose exceeding 65 Gy would be necessary to control 85% of subclinical disease [2].

Current guidelines of the European Association of Urology allow for selected PSC patients with ENE to be considered for adjuvant RT [11].

The other case in which adjuvant RT may be considered is in the case of positive pelvic lymph nodes. Data under these circumstances are even rarer than in the groin. Franks and colleagues described 23 PSC patients receiving RT to groin or pelvis [6]. Unfortunately, the cadre was sufficiently diverse that the only finding was relatively banal: patients receiving adjuvant RT had a greater overall survival than those receiving palliative RT ($p < 0.001$). In our multi-institutional analysis [12], adjuvant pelvic RT provided a 2.4-month improvement in median time to recurrence, a 4-month better median overall survival, and a 6-month better median disease-specific survival in patients with positive pelvic lymph nodes after pelvic dissection (Fig. 9.1). These benefits persisted in multivariable analysis.

In further proof that extrapolation from VuC or OPC to PSC is risky, randomized data in these diseases postoperatively reveal significant benefit, with hazard ratios of 0.45 ($p = 0.015$) for adjuvant RT in the former [13] and 0.75 ($p = 0.04$) for adjuvant chemoradiation in the latter [14].

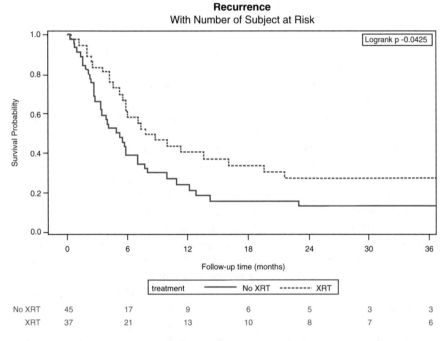

Fig. 9.1 Kaplan-Meier curve for recurrence-free survival in patients who received adjuvant pelvic radiation (XRT) vs. no radiation. (From Ref. [12]; used by permission)

Perioperative Chemotherapy

Inguinal lymph node involvement is an adverse prognostic factor in patients with penile carcinoma. Indeed, patients harboring uni- or bilateral inguinal lymph nodes (N1/N2), metastatic lymph node disease is highly likely. Similarly, presence of bulky or fixed inguinal lymphadenopathy (N3) uniformly signifies metastatic disease. In these clinical scenarios, perioperative chemotherapy is commonly advised to consolidate the effect of inguinal lymph node dissection, and to decrease the risk of regional or distant recurrence [15].

Neoadjuvant Chemotherapy

The European Association of Urology and the National Comprehensive Cancer

Network guidelines agree to recommend neoadjuvant chemotherapy in combination with radical inguinal ± pelvic lymph node dissection in patients with multiple, fixed, or bulky inguinal lymph nodes [16, 17]. Among the few pioneering studies investigating the use of neoadjuvant chemotherapy in patients with cN3 disease, Pizzocaro et al. [18] proved the benefit of neoadjuvant vincristine, bleomycin, and methotrexate showing a long-term survival in 37% of cases that achieved a complete response before surgery. Similarly, Leijte et al. [19] explored the effectiveness of five different chemotherapeutic regimens given preoperatively in 20 patients with advanced penile carcinoma. An objective tumor response was achieved in 12 (63%) of 19 evaluable patients. Overall, 5-yr survival was 32%. Lastly, Bermejo et al. [20] tested neoadjuvant chemotherapy in 59 patients with advanced penile carcinoma achieving stable, partial, or complete response in 10 (17%) patients. More recently, alternative chemotherapy regimens have been developed to increase the response rate. Nicholson et al. [21] tested the combination of docetaxel, cisplatin, and 5FU (TPF) in locally advanced or metastatic squamous carcinoma of the penis before surgery. Of all, 38.5% achieved a partial response. However, grade 3/4 adverse events were common in the treated population (65.5%), discouraging the routine use of TPF. The use of neoadjuvant chemotherapy has been also tested in patients with more confined lymph node disease (cN1–2). Here, the phase II study by Pagliaro et al. [22] evaluated the activity of the triple combination of paclitaxel, ifosfamide, and cisplatin (TIP) in patients with cN1–2 penile cancer. The investigators showed a 50% of objective response and 73% downstaged, which allowed consolidative surgery. The response to chemotherapy was significantly associated with both increased time to progression and overall survival. A recent systematic review and meta-analysis explored the benefit of neoadjuvant chemotherapy for locally advanced penile squamous cell carcinoma. Ten studies met the inclusion criteria, enrolling a total of 182 patients, with 66 (36.3%) and 116 (63.7%) treated with nontaxane-platinum and taxane-platinum regimens, respectively. The pooled findings in this study suggested that approximately half of the patients with bulky regional lymph node disease respond to platinum-based neoadjuvant chemotherapy, and approximately 16% of patients achieve a pathological complete response. Nontaxane-based regimens appear to be better tolerated than taxane regimens based on reported grade 3 or greater adverse events (26% vs 49%) [23]. Given the importance of local staging to differentiate among patients eligible and ineligible to neoadjuvant chemotherapy, Bandini et al. [24] developed a regression-tree prognostic tool that was able to identify patients who benefited from neoadjuvant chemotherapy among a cohort of 334 patients with cN+ disease. The authors found that patients with cN3 and cN2 with PET/CT-detected inguinal and pelvic nodal activity had lower probability to survive at 24 months, and thus they benefitted the most from neoadjuvant chemotherapy (hazard ratio 0.28, 95% confidence interval 0.13–0.62; $P = 0.002$). Taken together, TIP or TPF chemotherapy could be equally offered to patients with locally advanced penile carcinoma who are fit enough to tolerate combination regimens. Here, an appropriate staging carried with physical examination and PET/CT scan would help to select the right candidates.

Adjuvant Chemotherapy

The use of adjuvant chemotherapy in patients with nodal involvement is supported by European and American guidelines based on small and retrospective studies with heterogeneous study cohorts and/or subgroup analyses. To date, guidelines agree that adjuvant chemotherapy can be offered in pN2–3 after radical lymphadenectomy (LE: 2b). Instead, the use of adjuvant chemotherapy is not advised in low-risk patients (pN1–2). The first small retrospective study which supported adjuvant chemotherapy (vincristine, bleomycin, and methotrexate for 12 weeks) after radical inguino-pelvic resection in patients with locally advanced disease was published by Pizzocaro in 1988 [18]. This retrospective cohort included 12 patients with nodal metastases, of which nine had extra nodal extension, five had pelvic involvement, and five had bilateral metastasis. Only one patient relapsed after a follow-up of 18–102 months (median 42 months). The same group also published results of adjuvant chemotherapy with cisplatin, 5-FU plus paclitaxel or docetaxel (TPF), with three to four cycles after resection of pN2–3 disease. Here, among 19 patients, 52.6% were disease-free after a median follow-up of 42 months, with no severe side effects [25]. In 2015, Sharma et al. [26] compared overall survival between 36 patients who received adjuvant chemotherapy (different regimens) and 48 patients receiving observation. Median OS was 21.7 months (IQR: 11.8–104) in patients who received adjuvant chemotherapy vs. 10.1 (IQR: 5.6–48.1) in those who did not ($p = 0.048$). Beside the positive results of the study, it should be noted that the two cohorts were not uniformly balanced having younger patients with less aggressive penile tumor pathology, and less bilateral inguinal disease in the chemotherapy group. The only investigation that included patients with low-risk disease, namely, patients with stage pN1–2, was published by Necchi et al. in 2019 [27]. In this large retrospective study including over 700 patients, the sub-analysis on patients with pN1–2 diseases treated with or without adjuvant chemotherapy showed no benefit in favor of chemotherapy. Therefore, especially when taking into account the high morbidity of current chemotherapy regimens, adjuvant chemotherapy should not be given to low-risk patient.

Given the importance of tailoring the use of adjuvant treatments according with the risk of recurrence after surgery, prognostic models have given momentum. Recently, Bandini et al. [28] developed and externally validated a freely available risk calculator (https://marco-bandini-md-sanraffaele.shinyapps.io/PCRRC/) that predicts the probability of recurrence at 2 years from inguinal lymph node resection. Based on a large multi-institutional database, the authors identified 234 and 273 patients from development and validation cohorts, respectively, with $pT_{any}pN_{1-3} M_0$ disease that were treated with inguinal node dissection. According to the author's findings, positive surgical margins, pN3 status, and inguinal lymph node density were associated with higher recurrence rate. These factors were able to successfully stratify patients who did and did not benefit from adjuvant treatments (i.e., chemotherapy and/or radiotherapy). Taken together, adjuvant chemotherapy is advised in patients with high risk of progression after surgery. Here, the choice of the chemotherapeutic regimen and the duration of treatment should be tailored according to patient's tolerability.

Accessibility to Chemotherapy in Developing Countries

Penile carcinoma is a disease that presents heterogeneous geographical distribution. Developing countries such as South America, South Africa, and India report two to four times higher prevalence of patients affected by penile cancer compared with the rest of the world [29]. Unfortunately, treatment disparities are common in those areas of the globe where economic barriers hamper the use of expensive treatment modalities [30]. This phenomenon directly impacts on survival outcomes that are clearly in disadvantage in those countries where the access to cure is suboptimal [31]. Global effort should be spent to homogenize access to treatments in order to bring equal survival expectancy among patients from different geographical areas [32].

Role of HPV in Adjuvant Therapy of PSC

There is no doubt that concurrent HPV infection in OPC facilitates dose reduction of adjuvant RT [33]. The case for PSC is far less clear. In a review of our PSC patients with (+) lymph nodes between 1991 and 2016, adjuvant chemoradiation and HPV+ status were independently correlated with improved locoregional control. Similarly, in patients whose lesions were HPV (+), a locoregional control was only noted in those treated with adjuvant chemoradiation [34]. Similarly, in a large international database of PSC patients who had received inguinal lymph node dissection [35], patients with HPV+ lesions presented with lower clinical N stage ($p < 0.001$) and inguinal lymph node metastasis density ($p < 0.001$). Radiotherapy was more effective in the HPV+ subgroup, likely because of fewer TP53 mutations noted in that cadre.

However, in our genomic analysis of PSC, there was no difference in radiosensitivity between HPV-negative or HPV-positive lesions [2]. Thus, the question remains largely unresolved.

References

1. Yuan Z, Grass GD, Azizi M, Ahmed KA, Yoder GSJ, Welsh EA, Fulp WJ, Dhillon J, Torres-Roca JF, Giuliano AR, Spiess PE, Johnstone PAS. Intrinsic radiosensitivity, genomic-based radiation dose and patterns of failure of penile cancer in response to adjuvant radiation therapy. Rep Pract Oncol Radiother. 2019;24:593–9.

2. Yuan Z, Yang GQ, Ahmed KA, Torres-Roca JF, Spiess PE, Johnstone PAS. Radiation therapy in the management of the inguinal region in penile cancer: what's the evidence?. Urol Oncol Sem Orig Invest. 2020;S1078–1439(20)30198–8.
3. Ravi R, Chaturvedi HK, Sastry DV. Role of radiation therapy in the treatment of carcinoma of the penis. Br J Urol. 1994;74:646–51.
4. Graafland NM, Moonen LM, van Boven HH, et al. Inguinal recurrence following therapeutic lymphadenectomy for node positive penile carcinoma: outcome and implications for management. J Urol. 2011;185:888–93.
5. Burt LM, Shrieve DC, Tward JD. Stage presentation, care patterns, and treatment outcomes for squamous cell carcinoma of the penis. Int J Radiat Oncol Biol Phys. 2014;88:94–100.
6. Franks KN, Kancherla K, Sethugavalar B, et al. Radiotherapy for node positive penile cancer: experience of the Leeds teaching hospitals. J Urol. 2011;186:524–9.
7. Robinson R, Marconi L, MacPepple E, Hakenberg OW, Watkin N, Yuan Y, Lam T, MacLennan S, Adewuyi TE, Coscione A, Minhas SS, Compérat EM, Necchi A. Risks and benefits of adjuvant radiotherapy after inguinal lymphadenectomy in node-positive penile cancer: a systematic review by the European Association of Urology Penile Cancer Guidelines Panel. Eur Urol. 2018. pii: S0302–2838(18)30261–6. https://doi.org/10.1016/j.eururo.2018.04.003.
8. Chipollini J, Chaing S, Peyton CC, Sharma P, Kidd LC, Giuliano AR, Johnstone PA, Spiess PE. National Trends and Predictors of Locally Advanced Penile Cancer in the United States (1998-2012). Clin Genitourin Cancer. 2017;12:S1558–7673(17)30241–0. https://doi.org/10.1016/j.clgc.2017.07.031. Epub ahead of print.
9. Graafland NM, van Boven HH, van Werkhoven E, Moonen LM, Horenblas S. Prognostic significance of extranodal extension in patients with pathological node positive penile carcinoma. J Urol. 2010;184:1347–53.
10. Johnstone PAS, Boulware D, Ottenhof S, Djajadiningrat R, Necchi A, Catanzaro M, Ye D, Zhu Y, Nicolai N, Horenblas S, Spiess PE. Primary penile cancer: the role of adjuvant radiation therapy in management of extracapsular extension in lymph nodes. Eur Urol Focus. 2018;5(5):737–41. pii: S2405–4569(18)30300–6.
11. Hakenberg OW, Comperate EM, Minhas S, Necchi A, Protzel C, Watkin N. EAU guidelines on penile cancer: 2014 update. Eur Urol. 2015;67:152–50. Recent update?
12. Tang DH, Diorio G, Leone A, Schaible B, Ma Z, Djajadiningrat R, Catanzaro M, Ye D, Zhu Y, Nicolai N, Horenblas S, Johnstone PAS, Spiess PE. Adjuvant pelvic radiation is associated with improved overall survival and decreased disease recurrence in pelvic node-positive penile cancer after lymph node dissection: a multi-institutional study. Urol Oncol. 2017;35(10):605.e17–23.
13. Kunos C, Simpkins F, Gibbons H, et al. Radiation therapy compared with pelvic node resection for node-positive vulvar cancer: a randomized controlled trial. Obstet Gynecol. 2009;114:537.
14. Bernier J, Domenge C, Ozsahin M, et al. Postoperative irradiation with or without concomitant chemotherapy for locally advanced head and neck cancer. N Engl J Med. 2004;350:1945.
15. Bandini M, Pederzoli F, Necchi A. Neoadjuvant chemotherapy for lymph node-positive penile cancer: current evidence and knowledge. Curr Opin Urol. 2020;30(2):218–22.
16. Professionals S-O. EAU Guidelines: Penile Cancer [Internet]. Uroweb. [cited 2020 Mar 18]. Available from: https://uroweb.org/guideline/penile-cancer/.
17. Guidelines Detail [Internet]. [cited 2021 May 20]. Available from: https://www.nccn.org/guidelines/guidelines-detail?category=1&id=1456.
18. Pizzocaro G, Piva L. Adjuvant and neoadjuvant vincristine, bleomycin, and methotrexate for inguinal metastases from squamous cell carcinoma of the penis. Acta Oncol Stockh Swed. 1988;27(6b):823–4.
19. Leijte JAP, Kerst JM, Bais E, Antonini N, Horenblas S. Neoadjuvant chemotherapy in advanced penile carcinoma. Eur Urol. 2007;52(2):488–94.
20. Bermejo C, Busby JE, Spiess PE, Heller L, Pagliaro LC, Pettaway CA. Neoadjuvant chemotherapy followed by aggressive surgical consolidation for metastatic penile squamous cell carcinoma. J Urol. 2007;177(4):1335–8.

21. Nicholson S, Hall E, Harland SJ, Chester JD, Pickering L, Barber J, et al. Phase II trial of docetaxel, cisplatin and 5FU chemotherapy in locally advanced and metastatic penis cancer (CRUK/09/001). Br J Cancer. 2013;109(10):2554–9.
22. Pagliaro LC, Williams DL, Daliani D, Williams MB, Osai W, Kincaid M, et al. Neoadjuvant paclitaxel, ifosfamide, and cisplatin chemotherapy for metastatic penile cancer: a phase II study. J Clin Oncol Off J Am Soc Clin Oncol. 2010;28(24):3851–7.
23. Azizi M, Aydin AM, Hajiran A, Lai A, Kumar A, Peyton CC, et al. Systematic review and meta-analysis-is there a benefit in using neoadjuvant systemic chemotherapy for locally advanced penile squamous cell carcinoma? J Urol. 2020;203(6):1147–55.
24. Bandini M, Albersen M, Chipollini J, Pederzoli F, Zhu Y, Ye D-W, et al. Optimising the selection of candidates for neoadjuvant chemotherapy amongst patients with node-positive penile squamous cell carcinoma. BJU Int. 2020;125(6):867–75.
25. Survival analyses of adjuvant or neoadjuvant combination of a taxane plus cisplatin and 5-fluorouracil (T-PF) in patients with bulky nodal metastases from squamous cell carcinoma of the penis (PSCC): results of a single high-volume center. J Clin Oncol [Internet]. [cited 2021 May 20]. Available from: https://ascopubs.org/doi/abs/10.1200/jco.2014.32.4_suppl.377.
26. Sharma P, Djajadiningrat R, Zargar-Shoshtari K, Catanzaro M, Zhu Y, Nicolai N, et al. Adjuvant chemotherapy is associated with improved overall survival in pelvic node-positive penile cancer after lymph node dissection: a multi-institutional study. Urol Oncol. 2015;33(11): 496.e17–23.
27. Necchi A, Lo Vullo S, Mariani L, Zhu Y, Ye D-W, Ornellas AA, et al. Nomogram-based prediction of overall survival after regional lymph node dissection and the role of perioperative chemotherapy in penile squamous cell carcinoma: A retrospective multicenter study. Urol Oncol. 2019;37(8):531.e7–15.
28. Bandini M, Spiess PE, Pederzoli F, Marandino L, Brouwer OR, Albersen M, et al. A risk calculator predicting recurrence in lymph node metastatic penile cancer. BJU Int. 2020;126(5):577–85.
29. Thomas A, Necchi A, Muneer A, Tobias-Machado N, Tran ATH, Van Rompuy A-S, et al. Penile cancer. Nat Rev Dis Primer [Internet]. 2021 Feb 11 [cited 2021 May 20];7(1). Available from: https://pubmed.ncbi.nlm.nih.gov/33574340/.
30. Improving the Management of Rare Genitourinary Tumors Through International Collaborations: Together We Stand [Internet]. ASCO Daily News. [cited 2020 Dec 20]. Available from: https://doi.org/10.1200/ADN.20.200403/full.
31. Bandini M, Zhu Y, Ye D-W, Ornellas AA, Watkin N, Ayres B, et al. Contemporary treatment patterns and outcomes for patients with penile squamous cell carcinoma: identifying management gaps to promote multi-institutional collaboration. Eur Urol Oncol. 2020; 4(1):121–3.
32. Necchi A, Pederzoli F, Bandini M, Spiess PE. Revolutionizing care for rare genitourinary tumours. Nat Rev Urol. 2020;18(2):69–70.
33. Mesía R, Taberna M. HPV-related oropharyngeal carcinoma de-escalation protocols. Lancet Oncol. 2017;18(6):704–5.
34. Yuan Z, Naghavi AO, Tang D, Kim Y, Ahmed KA, Dhillon J, Giuliano A, Spiess PE, Johnstone PAS. The effect of HPV status and chemoradiotherapy in the management of pathologically node positive penile cancer. World J Urol. 2018;36(9):1431–40.
35. Bandini M, Ross JS, Zhu Y,Ye DW, Ornellas AA, Watkin N, Ayres BA, Hakenberg OW, Heidenreich A, Raggi D, Giannatempo P, Marandino L, Haidl F, Pederzoli F, Briganti A, Montorsi F, Chipollini J, Azizi M, De Meerleer G, Brouwer OR, Grass GD, Johnstone PA, Albersen M, Spiess PE, Necchi A. Association between human papillomavirus (HPV) infection and outcome of perioperative nodal radiotherapy for penile carcinoma. Eur Urol Oncol. (In press).

Chapter 10
Management of Locally Recurrent Penile Cancer

Alice Yu

Local Recurrence

Introduction

Penile sparing treatment (PST) should be considered in patients with noninvasive or minimally invasive tumors (Tis, Ta, T1). It presents several benefits over amputation, including preservation of penile length, glans sensation, and sexual quality of life without compromising long-term survival outcomes. Treatment options include topical therapy, laser treatment, radiation therapy, Mohs surgery, or wide local excision.

Local recurrence rates are higher compared to partial or total penectomy, and close follow-up is necessary. However, recurrence is not associated with worse cancer-specific or overall survival. Recurrence rates after PST can vary depending on the type of primary treatment, as well as the grade and stage of the primary tumor. Management of recurrent tumors typically involves surgical excision, though repeat PST can be offered in select cases.

Topical Therapy

Topical therapy with 5-fluorouracil (5-FU) or imiquimod is a treatment option for patients with noninvasive disease, particularly carcinoma in situ (CIS). A retrospective study of 45 patients who underwent topical therapy (5-FU or imiquimod) for

A. Yu (✉)
Department of Genitourinary Oncology, Moffitt Cancer Center, Tampa, FL, USA
e-mail: Alice.Yu@moffitt.org

© The Author(s), under exclusive license to Springer Nature Switzerland AG 2021   117
P. E. Spiess, A. Necchi (eds.), *Penile Carcinoma*,
https://doi.org/10.1007/978-3-030-82060-2_10

CIS of the penis showed a 57% complete response (CR) rate including 13.6% who experienced a partial response (PR) and 29.5% who experienced no response [1]. 20% of those who achieved CR developed a recurrence within 34 months median follow-up, highlighting the importance of continued surveillance after topical treatment.

Similarly, another series of 19 patients treated with 5-FU for 3 to 7 weeks for glandular CIS showed a 73.7% CR rate. All nonresponders underwent wide local excision or glansectomy and two out of five patients had pT1 on final pathology [2]. Thus, it is important to note that incomplete response to topical therapy may be a sign of undetected invasive disease, and treatment should not be repeated. In the setting of partial response or recurrence, surgical management in the form of wide local excision, glansectomy, partial or total penectomy should be considered.

Laser Treatment

Laser therapy has been used for the treatment of penile tumors (Tis, Ta, T1 G1–2) with acceptable outcomes. Four types of lasers have been described including carbon dioxide, Nd:YAG, argon, and potassium titanyl phosphate (KTP).

One review of 224 patients with Tis or T1 treated with carbon dioxide laser reported a 10-year recurrence rate of 17.5%, and a 10-year amputation rate of 5.5% [3]. Most cases of recurrence were treated with laser conservation excision, and two underwent amputation upfront. Seven patients recurred after salvage laser therapy and eventually required amputation. A subsequent study of 56 patients with T1 disease reported 13 (23%) local recurrences. The risk of recurrence increased with positive surgical margins and greater depth of invasion [4].

Radiation Therapy

External beam radiation therapy (EBRT) or brachytherapy are good options for patients with small (<4 cm), T1-T2 tumors. The American Brachytherapy Society and European Society of Therapeutic Radiation Oncology consensus statement for penile brachytherapy reported good tumor control rates, acceptable morbidity, and functional organ preservation for penile brachytherapy [5].

Local recurrence after radiation is typically salvaged with surgery. A retrospective review of 76 patients with predominant T1-T2 disease who underwent high-dose-rate brachytherapy reported a failure rate of 28.9%. This includes 8 (10.5%) cases of persistent disease and 14 (18.4%) cases of local recurrence. The median time to recurrence was 24 months (range 9–54 months) [6]. Patients with persistent disease or local recurrence were treated with penectomy except in four patients who refused surgery and underwent a second course of radiation therapy. There were no Grade 3 or 4 acute toxicities in this series. Only one case of urethral stenosis was observed, and it was treated successfully with dilatation. Distant metastases occurred in 12/76 (15.8%) cases. Five- and 10-year cancer-specific survival were 85.0% and 77.8%, respectively.

Radiation therapy is a good option for T1-T2 disease, and any recurrences can be salvaged with surgery. While penectomy provides better local control, there is no survival benefit [7].

Mohs Surgery

Mohs surgery is an alternative to wide local excision in select cases. Thin layers of cancerous skin are excised and examined microscopically until the tissue margin is negative for tumor. This allows for increased precision and preserves maximal tissue integrity. The success rate of Mohs surgery declines with higher staged diseases. One retrospective review of 33 patients (25 with follow-up) reported local recurrence in 8 (32%) patients after a mean follow-up of 58 months [8]. This series included tumor stages Tis to T3. Five cases were terminated with positive margins due to urethra involvement or large post-Mohs defect size. Seven out of eight recurrences were successfully managed by repeat Mohs surgery, and one patient with T3 disease required penectomy. One patient developed metastasis and died of the disease.

Thus, Mohs surgery seems to offer adequate local control and does not appear to impact overall survival. Local recurrences can be salvaged with additional Mohs surgery, particularly for small, superficial tumors where complete excision with negative margins is achievable.

Glansectomy and Wide Local Excision

Glansectomy can be considered for patients with distal tumors on the glans where removal of the glans alone can achieve a negative surgical margin. A retrospective study of 177 patients who underwent glansectomy with split-thickness skin graft reported a 9.3% local recurrence rate, and the median time to recurrence was 8.7 months [9]. On final surgical pathology, 32% had pT1, 56% had pT2 and 21% had pT3 disease. Cancer-specific mortality was 10.7% over a median time of 41.4 months. In this cohort, there were 17 cases of positive surgical margin on the final surgical specimen. Ten underwent revision surgery due to high-risk features at the resection margin. Seven had minimal margin involvement and negative frozen section; therefore, they were managed conservatively with close surveillance. One of the seven patients experienced local recurrence, and one of the ten men who underwent revision surgery developed local recurrence. Overall, glansectomy offers good local cancer control and functional outcomes [10, 11] and should be considered for distal tumors on the glans.

Wide local excision involves complete excision of the skin with or without skin graft. Superficial tumors on the penile shaft may be treated with wide local excision, and studies have shown that surgical margins of 5–10 mm are as safe and provide adequate tumor control [12]. Local recurrence is typically treated with partial or total penectomy.

Locally Advanced Disease

In patients with locally advanced recurrence, neoadjuvant chemotherapy (NAC) should be considered prior to surgical resection. In a meta-analysis of 10 studies and 182 patients treated with perioperative NAC, an objective response was observed in 53% of patients. In addition, pathologic complete response was seen in 16% [13].

Summary

Tis, Ta, and T1 penile cancer can be managed with conservative, organ-sparing approaches without impacting long-term survival outcomes. Several studies comparing PST to partial or total penectomy have shown no difference in regional recurrence, metastasis-free survival, or overall survival [14–16]. However, patients treated with PST have a significantly higher risk of local recurrence (28%) compared to those treated with amputation (5%) [17]. Patient compliance with follow-up needs to be considered since close surveillance is critical for early detection and treatment.

Recurrent tumors should be treated based on the tumor location, size, and stage. Non-invasive recurrence (Tis or Ta) is often managed with surgical resection, although repeat PST can be considered. Patients with invasive disease at time of recurrence should undergo partial or total penectomy.

Regional Recurrence

Regional Recurrence Without Primary ILND

There is evidence that patients with high-risk penile tumors have better survival outcomes with immediate ILND rather than delayed ILND [18, 19]. Patients who have lower-risk tumors or those with high-risk disease who refuse immediate ILND must undergo surveillance and may experience an inguinal nodal recurrence during follow-up. A retrospective review of 395 patients with cN0 disease who did not undergo immediate ILND found a 9% regional recurrence rate. Over 85% of recurrences transpired within the first 2 years and 100% occurred within the first 5 years of follow-up [17].

In patients without prior inguinal lymphadenectomy or radiation, primary treatment of the inguinal lymph nodes with surgery or radiation should be considered. Treatment should be based on exam characteristics such as number, size, and mobility of the lymph node (Fig. 10.1). Solitary mobile nodes that are <4 cm should be biopsied, and if positive, treated with ILND.

Bulky lymphadenopathy that is >4 cm, fixed or multi-nodal should be treated with neoadjuvant chemotherapy once biopsy is proven positive. Patients who respond well to chemotherapy should undergo inguinal and pelvic lymph node dissection or RT.

Regional Recurrence After Primary ILND

Inguinal lymph node dissection (ILND) is recommended for invasive primary disease or palpable lymph nodes at presentation and cure rates can be as high as 80% in patients with one or two involved lymph nodes without extranodal extension (ENE) [20–23]. A retrospective study of 700 patients treated at two European centers showed that in patients surgically staged as pN0, the regional recurrence rate is 2%, compared to 19% in those with N+ disease [17]. Patients with three or more positive nodes, ENE, or pelvic lymphadenopathy are at particularly high risk of regional recurrence [24, 25].

Most inguinal recurrences occur after a median of 5–7 months from the initial lymph node dissection [24–26]. These cases carry an especially poor prognosis with a median survival of <6 months [24, 25]. In the absence of high-level evidence, the role of adjuvant chemotherapy or RT is controversial. We hope that the upcoming International Penile Advanced Cancer Trial (InPACT) may help address some of these questions.

Patients with inguinal recurrence are at high risk of metastatic progression. It is important to rule out disseminated disease before proceeding with aggressive multimodal treatment. There is emerging data suggesting that PET/CT has good sensitivity for M staging [27]. Especially in patients with inguinal lymphadenopathy, sensitivity for pelvic lymph node metastasis is 91–93% [28].

If the patient previously received lymphadenectomy or RT, salvage options include chemotherapy followed by ILND, ILND alone, or chemoradiation, if there was no history of prior RT (Fig. 10.1).

For appropriately selected patients, salvage ILND can be considered. A retrospective review of 20 patients who underwent salvage ILND with curative intent showed a median CSS of 16.4 months (95% CI 5.1–27.8) with 9 (45%) patients having no evidence of disease (NED) at 12 months [26]. A median of 3 (range 1–17) lymph nodes were resected at the time of salvage ILND and a median of 2 (range 1–7) lymph nodes were positive for malignancy. Of note, 12 (60%) patients received adjuvant chemotherapy and 2 (10%) received adjuvant RT. Postoperative complications included wound infection in six patients (30%), severe debilitating lymphedema in 4 (20%), and a seroma in one patient that resolved with percutaneous aspiration [26].

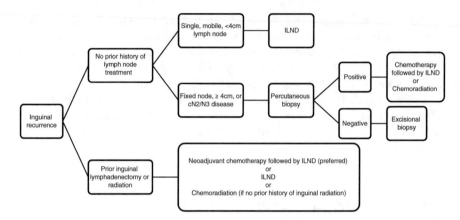

Fig. 10.1 Management of inguinal recurrence. ILND: inguinal lymph node dissection

Salvage surgery has been fraught with high morbidity and often requires reconstructive flaps [29]. One study of 15 patients with advanced locoregional disease underwent local surgical resection with Rectus abdominis myocutaneous or abdominal advancement flap reconstruction. Thirteen of the 15 patients (87%) experienced wound complications, including five Clavien-Dindo grade III complications [29].

Another series reported 26 patients who developed inguinal recurrence after primary ILND. Salvage treatment included surgery, inguinal RT, chemotherapy, chemoradiation, and no treatment [24]. Two patients underwent salvage ILND, including one after induction chemotherapy. Of those two patients, one died of unrelated causes 10 years after treatment and the other was alive and NED at 16 months. The remaining 24 patients died of disease within 14 months of recurrence [24].

Summary

Patients with regional recurrence with no previous ILND should be treated in the same way as patients with primary inguinal lymphadenopathy. Patients with regional lymph node recurrence after prior lymphadenectomy have disrupted inguinal lymphatic drainage and are at a high risk of metastatic progression. PET/CT may help rule out disseminated disease before proceeding with therapy [27]. As for treatment options, the best quality data supports use of NAC followed by salvage ILND [24, 26].

References

1. Alnajjar HM, Lam W, Bolgeri M, Rees RW, Perry MJ, Watkin NA. Treatment of carcinoma in situ of the glans penis with topical chemotherapy agents. Eur Urol. 2012;62(5):923–8.

2. Lucky M, Murthy KV, Rogers B, Jones S, Lau MW, Sangar VK, et al. The treatment of penile carcinoma in situ (CIS) within a UK supra-regional network. BJU Int. 2015;115(4): 595–8.
3. Bandieramonte G, Colecchia M, Mariani L, Lo Vullo S, Pizzocaro G, Piva L, et al. Peniscopically controlled CO2 laser excision for conservative treatment of in situ and T1 penile carcinoma: report on 224 patients. Eur Urol. 2008;54(4):875–82.
4. Colecchia M, Nicolai N, Secchi P, Bandieramonte G, Paganoni AM, Sangalli LM, et al. pT1 penile squamous cell carcinoma: a clinicopathologic study of 56 cases treated by CO2 laser therapy. Anal Quant Cytol Histol. 2009;31(3):153–60.
5. Crook JM, Haie-Meder C, Demanes DJ, Mazeron JJ, Martinez AA, Rivard MJ. American Brachytherapy Society-Groupe Europeen de Curietherapie-European Society of Therapeutic Radiation Oncology (ABS-GEC-ESTRO) consensus statement for penile brachytherapy. Brachytherapy. 2013;12(3):191–8.
6. Kellas-Sleczka S, Bialas B, Fijalkowski M, Wojcieszek P, Szlag M, Cholewka A, et al. Nineteen-year single-center experience in 76 patients with penile cancer treated with high-dose-rate brachytherapy. Brachytherapy. 2019;18(4):493–502.
7. Hasan S, Francis A, Hagenauer A, Hirsh A, Kaminsky D, Traughber B, et al. The role of brachytherapy in organ preservation for penile cancer: a meta-analysis and review of the literature. Brachytherapy. 2015;14(4):517–24.
8. Shindel AW, Mann MW, Lev RY, Sengelmann R, Petersen J, Hruza GJ, et al. Mohs micrographic surgery for penile cancer: management and long-term followup. J Urol. 2007; 178(5):1980–5.
9. Parnham AS, Albersen M, Sahdev V, Christodoulidou M, Nigam R, Malone P, et al. Glansectomy and split-thickness skin graft for penile cancer. Eur Urol. 2018; 73(2):284–9.
10. O'Kane HF, Pahuja A, Ho KJ, Thwaini A, Nambirajan T, Keane P. Outcome of glansectomy and skin grafting in the management of penile cancer. Adv Urol. 2011;2011:240824.
11. Morelli G, Pagni R, Mariani C, Campo G, Menchini-Fabris F, Minervini R, et al. Glansectomy with split-thickness skin graft for the treatment of penile carcinoma. Int J Impot Res. 2009;21(5):311–4.
12. Minhas S, Kayes O, Hegarty P, Kumar P, Freeman A, Ralph D. What surgical resection margins are required to achieve oncological control in men with primary penile cancer? BJU Int. 2005;96(7):1040–3.
13. Azizi M, Aydin AM, Hajiran A, Lai A, Kumar A, Peyton CC, et al. Systematic review and meta-analysis-is there a benefit in using neoadjuvant systemic chemotherapy for locally advanced penile squamous cell carcinoma? J Urol. 2020;203(6):1147–55.
14. Lindner AK, Schachtner G, Steiner E, Kroiss A, Uprimny C, Steinkohl F, et al. Organ-sparing surgery of penile cancer: higher rate of local recurrence yet no impact on overall survival. World J Urol. 2020;38(2):417–24.
15. Djajadiningrat RS, van Werkhoven E, Meinhardt W, van Rhijn BW, Bex A, van der Poel HG, et al. Penile sparing surgery for penile cancer-does it affect survival? J Urol. 2014; 192(1):120–5.
16. Kamel MH, Tao J, Su J, Khalil MI, Bissada NK, Schurhamer B, et al. Survival outcomes of organ sparing surgery, partial penectomy, and total penectomy in pathological T1/T2 penile cancer: Report from the National Cancer Data Base. Urol Oncol. 2018;36(2):82.e7–15.
17. Leijte JA, Kirrander P, Antonini N, Windahl T, Horenblas S. Recurrence patterns of squamous cell carcinoma of the penis: recommendations for follow-up based on a two-centre analysis of 700 patients. Eur Urol. 2008;54(1):161–8.
18. Kroon BK, Horenblas S, Lont AP, Tanis PJ, Gallee MP, Nieweg OE. Patients with penile carcinoma benefit from immediate resection of clinically occult lymph node metastases. J Urol. 2005;173(3):816–9.
19. McDougal WS. Preemptive lymphadenectomy markedly improves survival in patients with cancer of the penis who harbor occult metastases. J Urol. 2005;173(3):681.

20. Horenblas S, van Tinteren H, Delemarre JF, Moonen LM, Lustig V, van Waardenburg EW. Squamous cell carcinoma of the penis. III. Treatment of regional lymph nodes. J Urol. 1993;149(3):492–7.
21. Ravi R. Correlation between the extent of nodal involvement and survival following groin dissection for carcinoma of the penis. Br J Urol. 1993;72(5 Pt 2):817–9.
22. Graafland NM, van Boven HH, van Werkhoven E, Moonen LM, Horenblas S. Prognostic significance of extranodal extension in patients with pathological node positive penile carcinoma. J Urol. 2010;184(4):1347–53.
23. Lont AP, Kroon BK, Gallee MP, van Tinteren H, Moonen LM, Horenblas S. Pelvic lymph node dissection for penile carcinoma: extent of inguinal lymph node involvement as an indicator for pelvic lymph node involvement and survival. J Urol. 2007;177(3):947–52. discussion 52.
24. Graafland NM, Moonen LM, van Boven HH, van Werkhoven E, Kerst JM, Horenblas S. Inguinal recurrence following therapeutic lymphadenectomy for node positive penile carcinoma: outcome and implications for management. J Urol. 2011;185(3):888–93.
25. Reddy JP, Pettaway CA, Levy LB, Pagliaro LC, Tamboli P, Rao P, et al. Factors associated with regional recurrence after lymph node dissection for penile squamous cell carcinoma. BJU Int. 2017;119(4):591–7.
26. Baumgarten AS, Alhammali E, Hakky TS, Espiritu PN, Pow-Sang JM, Sexton WJ, et al. Salvage surgical resection for isolated locally recurrent inguinal lymph node metastasis of penile cancer: international study collaboration. J Urol. 2014;192(3):760–4.
27. Ottenhof SR, Leone AR, Horenblas S, Spiess PE, Vegt E. Advancements in staging and imaging for penile cancer. Curr Opin Urol. 2017;27(6):612–20.
28. Ottenhof SR, Vegt E. The role of PET/CT imaging in penile cancer. Transl Androl Urol. 2017;6(5):833–8.
29. Ottenhof SR, Leone A, Djajadiningrat RS, Azizi M, Zargar K, Kidd LC, et al. Surgical and oncological outcomes in patients after vascularised flap reconstruction for Locoregionally advanced penile cancer. Eur Urol Focus. 2019;5(5):867–74.

Chapter 11
Management of Metastatic Penile Cancer

Bradley A. McGregor and Guru P. Sonpavde

Introduction

Penile squamous cell carcinoma (PSCC) is an orphan malignancy that comprises <1% of all cancers in men in the United States, with only approximately 2200 new cases per year coupled with 500 deaths annually [1]. However, in other parts of the world including South Asia, South America, and Africa, PSCC accounts for up to 20% of malignancies in men [2, 3]. Unfortunately, once the patient develops metastatic disease, prognosis remains poor with a median survival less than 1 year and 5 year overall survival (OS) of 5–10% [4]. This chapter reviews systemic chemotherapy for advanced PSCC.

Front-Line Treatment Regimens

Platinum-based chemotherapy remains the mainstay of systemic therapy for metastatic PSCC based on several single-arm phase 2 trials in the neoadjuvant and metastatic setting (Table 11.1). Cisplatin was first studied in a cooperative group trial showing an ORR of 15.4% with single-agent therapy [5]. Small case series of cisplatin in combination with methotrexate, and interferon led to further combination trials [6, 7]. The first triplet trial actually explored a nonplatinum regimen with vincristine, bleomycin, and methotrexate with objective responses in three of five

B. A. McGregor · G. P. Sonpavde (✉)
Lank Center for Genitourinary Oncology, Dana Farber Cancer Institute and Harvard Medical School, Boston, MA, USA
e-mail: Bradley_McGregor@DFCI.HARVARD.EDU; gurup_sonpavde@dfci.harvard.edu

© The Author(s), under exclusive license to Springer Nature Switzerland AG 2021   125
P. E. Spiess, A. Necchi (eds.), *Penile Carcinoma*,
https://doi.org/10.1007/978-3-030-82060-2_11

Table 11.1 Front-line regimens utilized in treatment of metastatic penile carcinoma

Platinum	Additional medications	Cycle length	Data source	ORR
Cisplatin 25 mg/m² D1–3	Ifosfamide 1200 mg/m² D1–3 Paclitaxel 175 mg/m² MESNA 400 mg/m² prior to ifosfamide and 200 mg/m² 4 and 8 hours later	21 days	Prospective, neoadjuvant	50% ($n = 15$) [10]
Cisplatin 80 mg/m² D1	Irinotecan 60 mg/m² D1,8, 15	28 days	Prospective	30.8% ($N = 28$) [13]
Cisplatin 70–80 mg/m² D1	Flourouracil 800– 100 mg/m² CI D1–4	21 days	Retrospective	32% ($n = 25$) [11]
Cisplatin 70 mg/m² D1	Docetaxel 75 mg/m² D1 Flourouracil 500 mg/m²/ day CI D1–5	21 days	Prospective	38.5% ($n = 39$) [12]
Cisplatin 75 mg/m² D1	Bleomycin 10 mg/m² D1,8 Methotrexate 20 mg/m² D1,8	21 days	Prospective	32.5% ($n = 40$) [9]
Carboplatin AUC 6	Paclitaxel 175 mg/m²	21 days	Retrospective	1 PR, 1 SD ($n = 2$) [14]
–	Dacomitnib 45 mg PO daily	–	Prospective	32.1% ($n = 28$) [16]

patients but two patients developed pulmonary fibrosis [8]. Combining cisplatin with bleomycin and methotrexate yielded encouraging responses in a trial of 45 patients with metastatic disease with five complete and eight partial responses among 40 evaluable patients for a 32.5% response rate. However, five treatment-related deaths occurred, and among the 36 remaining patients evaluable for toxicity, six patients had one or more life-threatening toxic episodes [9]. However, building upon the encouraging response rate other less toxic cisplatin-based regimens have been developed.

The mainstay of treatment in the metastatic setting is considered to be cisplatin in combination with ifosfamide and paclitaxel (TIP regimen) given data in the neo-adjuvant setting. In a trial of 30 patients who received neoadjuvant TIP for locally advanced disease, 15 (50.0%, (95% CI, 0.31 to 0.69)) exhibited an objective response with 3 complete responses (CRs) and 12 partial responses (PRs). Only six patients (20%) experienced progressive disease (PD) as best response. The regimen was well tolerated with manageable toxicities with no grade 4 events occurring in more than one patient to include grade 4 neutropenia. However, there were five episodes of grade 3 infections and, therefore, prophylactic granulocyte growth factor support is typically recommended [10].

Given the activity of combination cisplatin and 5-flourouracil (FU) in other squamous cell carcinomas, this regimen has been pursued; retrospective analyses have shown the activity in an analysis of 78 patients. PRs and stable disease (SD) were observed in eight (32%) and 10 (40%) patients, respectively, with a disease control rate (DCR) of 72%. However, median PFS was short at 20 weeks and median OS was only 8 months. Furthermore, this regimen was not without toxicity; grade 3 or 4 neutropenia was observed in 20% of patients with expected grade 1 toxicities of grade 1 or 2 neutropenia, oral mucositis and nausea/vomiting seen in 30–44% of patients [11]. In a study of 39 patients adding docetaxel to cisplatin and 5FU, the objective response rate (ORR) appeared slightly higher at 38.5% while the median OS was only 9 months with no CRs observed. Most common grade 3 or higher toxicities were neutropenia (33%), nausea/vomiting (18%). Overall, given the potential for CR with the TIP regimen, the cisplatin, 5FU, docetaxel regimen has not been widely adopted, and the older bleomycin-containing regimens have been abandoned due to pulmonary toxicities [12].

Other trials involving cisplatin combinations have been pursued with discouraging results. A trial examining the combination of cisplatin with irinotecan in 28 patients showed a modest ORR of 30.8%. Further studies of this regimen in the metastatic setting are not planned [13]. For those who are not eligible for cisplatin-based chemotherapy combination, carboplatin and taxol remains a viable option based on limited retrospective data. In an analysis of 59 treated patients with advanced penile carcinoma, only two patients received the combination of carboplatin with paclitaxel with one achieving a PR and the other stable disease [14]. A case report used the combination at dose of carboplatin AUC 3 and paclitaxel 75 mg/m^2 every 3 weeks with response [15].

There has been intriguing data with epidermal growth factor receptor (EGFR) inhibitors in this setting as well. Dacomitinib, an irreversible, pan-epidermal growth factor receptor inhibitor was studied in a single arm phase 2 study of 28 chemo naïve patients. One complete and eight partial responses were obtained (ORR 32.1%) with a 12-month PFS of 26.2% and 12-month OS of 54.9%. This was well tolerated though near 11% ($n = 3$) of patients experienced a grade 3 skin toxicity. Interestingly, there was no association of response with EGFR amplification though telomerase reverse transcriptase (TERT) mutations were found in responders only (60%), and phosphatidylinositol 3-kinase/mammalian target of rapamycin (PI3K/mTOR) pathway gene mutations were enriched in responders suggesting mutations in downstream effectors of EGFR signaling may sensitize to EGFR inhibition [16].

Second-Line Treatment Regimens

There is no standard second-line regimen following progression on a cisplatin-based regimen. In general, surgery is not effective; among 19 patients who relapsed following TIP, four patients underwent salvage surgery, all experienced further disease progression within 2 months [17]. In an analysis of 17 who went on to receive ≥1 salvage therapy following progression on TIP median OS from first treatment failure was 5.7 months (range, 1.4–30.3 months). Therapies received include cisplatin in combination with methotrexate and bleomycin, gemcitabine in combination with docetaxel or vinorelbine as well as cetuximab with cisplatin. Akin to data in the front-line setting, bleomycin, methotrexate, and cisplatin was active with objective responses in 2 of 5 patients including one CR though associated with significant toxicity; one patient developed fatal pneumonitis. There were no other documented responses to other systemic therapy. Of note, while there was a month improvement in PFS among those receiving additional cisplatin-based therapy (5.6 vs 4.2 months), this was not statistically significant ($p = 0.4$) [17].

In another analysis of 63 patients receiving a variety of chemotherapy in the post-platinum setting (48 received taxane therapy alone or in combination and 17 received cetuximab alone or in combination), 17 patients had a response (27.0%) and median OS and PFS were 20 and 12 weeks, respectively. Cetuximab-including regimens were associated with a trend for improved RR compared to other agents (odds ratio = 5.05, $p = 0.077$). Other analyses looking at taxanes vs. non-taxane, and combination vs. single agent therapy was not associated with improved outcomes [18].

Single-arm phase 2 trials have expanded on these retrospective analyses. In a single-arm multicenter phase 2 trials, 25 taxane-naïve patients were treated with 175 mg/m^2 paclitaxel at 3 week intervals until disease progression or irreversible toxicity. ORR was 20% though responses were short-lived with median PFS only 11 weeks and OS of 23 weeks. Toxicities were as expected with grade 1–2 neutropenia, nausea, and oral mucositis the most common side effects, noted in 13, 9, and 8 patients, respectively. Grade 3–4 neutropenia was reported in seven patients (28%) [19].

EGFR inhibitors may be considered reasonable, especially in those with genomic analysis of PSCC showing activating mutations in EGFR [20–23]. Case reports have shown activity of taxanes in combination with monoclonal antibodies targeting EGFR with acceptable toxicity [24]. In a retrospective analysis, 24 patients had received EGFR-targeted therapies, including cetuximab, erlotinib, and gefitinib. As expected, the most common adverse effect was skin rash (71%) [25]. Among 17 patients treated with cetuximab alone or in combination with cisplatin, there were four partial responses (23.5%) including two patients with seemingly chemo-resistant tumor. In this analysis, cetuximab had been given with a loading dose of 400 mg/m^2 on day 1 and then at 250 mg/m^2 weekly [25].

Largest set of prospective data involves a trial of 11 patients with chemo-refractory disease who received panitumumab 6 mg/kg every 2 weeks until disease progression or unacceptable toxicity. They noted one case of grade 3 cutaneous toxicity and diarrhea each, and two cases of grade 3 mucositis with one patient requiring discontinuation due to skin toxicity. ORR was 27% (2 CR, 1 PR); median PFS was 1.9 months and median OS was 9.5 months. The presence of visceral metastases showed a trend for association with worse OS ($P = 0.098$) [26]. Unfortunately, a similar trial exploring the use of afatinib in this setting was terminated due to poor accrual.

Recently, scant data have emerged demonstrating activity for immune checkpoint inhibitors at least in a subset of patients with metastatic PSCC harboring molecular vulnerabilities [27, 28]. It is noteworthy that pembrolizumab is approved by the US FDA for patients regardless of malignancy if the tumor mutation burden exceeds 10 mutations/megabase or for microsatellite instability (MSI)-high (H) tumors. In contrast, the combination of ipilimumab and nivolumab demonstrated no responses in a small-phase II trial across variant urologic malignancies [29].

Prognostic Factors in Metastatic Penile Carcinoma

Multiple retrospective analyses have analyzed prognostic markers in the setting of cytotoxic chemotherapy for penile carcinoma in the front- and second-line setting. In an analysis of 140 men with penile carcinoma of which nearly 75% received cisplatin-based chemotherapy, a multivariate model showed presence of visceral metastases and ECOG PS $\geq$ 1 to both be poor prognostic markers for progression-free survival (PFS) and overall survival (OS). Subsequently, a model was developed stratifying by the presence of neither, one, or both risk factors was developed. Median OS for the entire cohort was 9 months, while among those with no risk factors the median OS had not been reached while it was 8 and 7 months for those with one or both risk factors, respectively [4]. The 6-month OS decreased 92.4% to 76.1%, to 53.0%, with none, one or both risk factors. With even more separation at 1 year at 65.5% vs 9.6 and 13.3%. Notably, cisplatin-based regimens were associated with better OS though not PFS compared with non-cisplatin-based regimens after adjusting for presence of visceral metastases and performance status [4]. Other analyses have also shown presence of bone metastases to be a poor prognostic marker while younger age, longer time to recurrence and lower histological grade were associated with longer PFS and OS [11, 25].

In the second-line setting, following platinum-based therapy, visceral metastasis and depressed hemoglobin ($\leq$10 gm/dl) were both associated with poor overall survival in a retrospective analysis. Among those patients with neither risk factor, the median OS was 24 weeks and 1-year OS was 13.7%. However, with low hemoglobin and/or presence of visceral metastases, median overall survival was only 20 weeks; 1-year OS was nearly half at 6.7% [18].

Current Recommendations

At this time, the standard of care for metastatic penile carcinoma remains a cisplatin-based combination with TIP preferred. Following progression on platinum-based therapy, EGFR-targeted therapies or trials may be pursued. Pembrolizumab is formally approved for patients harboring any malignancy with the MSI-H profile or $\geq$10 mutations/megabase. Studies exploring the molecular biology of penile carcinoma will be critical to advancing the care for these patients to provide rational therapeutic advances while advancing precision medicine [20].

Disclosures

Bradley A. McGregor:

- Consulting: Bayer, Astellas, AstraZeneca, Seattle Genetics, Exelixis, Nektar, Pfizer, Janssen, Genentech, Eisai, Dendreon, Bristol-Myers Squibb and EMD Serono.
- Research support for the Dana-Farber Cancer Institute from Bristol-Myers Squibb, Calithera, Exelixis, and Seattle Genetics.

Guru P. Sonpavde:

- Advisory Board: BMS, Genentech, EMD Serono, Merck, Sanofi, Seattle Genetics/Astellas, Astrazeneca, Exelixis, Janssen, Bicycle Therapeutics, Pfizer, Immunomedics.
- Research Support to Institution: Sanofi, Astrazeneca, Immunomedics.
- Travel costs: BMS, Astrazeneca.
- Speaking fees: Physicians Education Resource (PER), Onclive, Research to Practice, Medscape.
- Writing fees: Uptodate, Editor of Elsevier Practice Update Bladder Cancer Center of Excellence.
- Steering committee of trials/studies: BMS, Bavarian Nordic, Seattle Genetics, QED (all unpaid), and Astrazeneca, EMD Serono, Debiopharm (paid).

References

1. Howlader N, Noone AM, Krapcho M, Miller D, Brest A, Yu M, Ruhl J, Tatalovich Z, Mariotto A, Lewis DR, Chen HS, Feuer EJ, Cronin KA, editors. SEER Cancer Statistics Review, 1975–2017, National Cancer Institute. Bethesda, MD, https://seer.cancer.gov/csr/1975_2017/, based on November 2019 SEER data submission, posted to the SEER web site, April 2020.
2. Ornellas AA. Management of penile cancer. J Surg Oncol. 2008;97(3):199–200.
3. Siegel RL, Miller KD, Fuchs HE, Jemal A. Cancer statistics, 2021. CA Cancer J Clin. 2021;71(1):7–33.
4. Pond GR, Di Lorenzo G, Necchi A, Eigl BJ, Kolinsky MP, Chacko RT, et al. Prognostic risk stratification derived from individual patient level data for men with advanced penile squamous cell carcinoma receiving first-line systemic therapy. Urol Oncol. 2014;32(4):501–8.
5. Gagliano RG, Blumenstein BA, Crawford ED, Stephens RL, Coltman CA Jr, Costanzi JJ. cis-Diamminedichloroplatinum in the treatment of advanced epidermoid carcinoma of the penis: a Southwest Oncology Group Study. J Urol. 1989;141(1):66–7.
6. Kattan J, Culine S, Droz JP, Fadel E, Court B, Perrin JL, et al. Penile cancer chemotherapy: twelve years' experience at Institut Gustave-Roussy. Urology. 1993;42(5):559–62.
7. Mitropoulos D, Dimopoulos MA, Kiroudi-Voulgari A, Zervas A, Dimopoulos C, Logothetis CJ. Neoadjuvant cisplatin and interferon-alpha 2B in the treatment and organ preservation of penile carcinoma. J Urol. 1994;152(4):1124–6.
8. Pizzocaro G, Piva L. Adjuvant and neoadjuvant vincristine, bleomycin, and methotrexate for inguinal metastases from squamous cell carcinoma of the penis. Acta Oncol (Stockholm, Sweden). 1988;27(6b):823–4.

9. Haas GP, Blumenstein BA, Gagliano RG, Russell CA, Rivkin SE, Culkin DJ, et al. Cisplatin, methotrexate and bleomycin for the treatment of carcinoma of the penis: a Southwest Oncology Group study. J Urol. 1999;161(6):1823–5.
10. Pagliaro LC, Williams DL, Daliani D, Williams MB, Osai W, Kincaid M, et al. Neoadjuvant paclitaxel, ifosfamide, and cisplatin chemotherapy for metastatic penile cancer: a phase II study. J Clin Oncol. 2010;28(24):3851–7.
11. Di Lorenzo G, Buonerba C, Federico P, Perdonà S, Aieta M, Rescigno P, et al. Cisplatin and 5-fluorouracil in inoperable, stage IV squamous cell carcinoma of the penis. BJU Int. 2012;110(11 Pt B):E661–6.
12. Zhang S, Zhu Y, Ye D. Phase II study of docetaxel, cisplatin, and fluorouracil in patients with distantly metastatic penile cancer as first-line chemotherapy. Oncotarget. 2015; 6(31):32212–9.
13. Theodore C, Skoneczna I, Bodrogi I, Leahy M, Kerst JM, Collette L, et al. A phase II multicentre study of irinotecan (CPT 11) in combination with cisplatin (CDDP) in metastatic or locally advanced penile carcinoma (EORTC PROTOCOL 30992). Ann Oncol. 2008; 19(7):1304–7.
14. Bermejo C, Busby JE, Spiess PE, Heller L, Pagliaro LC, Pettaway CA. Neoadjuvant chemotherapy followed by aggressive surgical consolidation for metastatic penile squamous cell carcinoma. J Urol. 2007;177(4):1335–8.
15. Joerger M, Warzinek T, Klaeser B, Kluckert JT, Schmid HP, Gillessen S. Major tumor regression after paclitaxel and carboplatin polychemotherapy in a patient with advanced penile cancer. Urology. 2004;63(4):778–80.
16. Necchi A, Lo Vullo S, Perrone F, Raggi D, Giannatempo P, Calareso G, et al. First-line therapy with dacomitinib, an orally available pan-HER tyrosine kinase inhibitor, for locally advanced or metastatic penile squamous cell carcinoma: results of an open-label, single-arm, single-centre, phase 2 study. BJU Int. 2018;121(3):348–56.
17. Wang J, Pettaway CA, Pagliaro LC. Treatment for metastatic penile cancer after first-line chemotherapy failure: analysis of response and survival outcomes. Urology. 2015; 85(5):1104–10.
18. Buonerba C, Di Lorenzo G, Pond G, Cartenì G, Scagliarini S, Rozzi A, et al. Prognostic and predictive factors in patients with advanced penile cancer receiving salvage (2nd or later line) systemic treatment: a retrospective, multi-center study. Front Pharmacol. 2016;7:487.
19. Di Lorenzo G, Federico P, Buonerba C, Longo N, Cartenì G, Autorino R, et al. Paclitaxel in pretreated metastatic penile cancer: final results of a phase 2 study. Eur Urol. 2011; 60(6):1280–4.
20. Feber A, Worth DC, Chakravarthy A, de Winter P, Shah K, Arya M, et al. CSN1 somatic mutations in penile squamous cell carcinoma. Cancer Res. 2016;76(16):4720–7.
21. McDaniel AS, Hovelson DH, Cani AK, Liu CJ, Zhai Y, Zhang Y, et al. Genomic profiling of penile squamous cell carcinoma reveals new opportunities for targeted therapy. Cancer Res. 2015;75(24):5219–27.
22. Ali SM, Pal SK, Wang K, Palma NA, Sanford E, Bailey M, et al. Comprehensive genomic profiling of advanced penile carcinoma suggests a high frequency of clinically relevant genomic alterations. Oncologist. 2016;21(1):33–9.
23. Jacob JM, Ferry EK, Gay LM, Elvin JA, Vergilio JA, Ramkissoon S, et al. Comparative genomic profiling of refractory and metastatic penile and nonpenile cutaneous squamous cell carcinoma: implications for selection of systemic therapy. J Urol. 2019;201(3):541–8.
24. Rescigno P, Matano E, Raimondo L, Mainolfi C, Federico P, Buonerba C, et al. Combination of docetaxel and cetuximab for penile cancer: a case report and literature review. Anti-Cancer Drugs. 2012;23(5):573–7.
25. Carthon BC, Ng CS, Pettaway CA, Pagliaro LC. Epidermal growth factor receptor-targeted therapy in locally advanced or metastatic squamous cell carcinoma of the penis. BJU Int. 2014;113(6):871–7.

26. Necchi A, Giannatempo P, Lo Vullo S, Raggi D, Nicolai N, Colecchia M, et al. Panitumumab treatment for advanced penile squamous cell carcinoma when surgery and chemotherapy have failed. Clin Genitourin Cancer. 2016;14(3):231–6.
27. Chahoud J, Skelton WP, Spiess PE, Walko C, Dhillon J, Gage KL, et al. Case report: two cases of chemotherapy refractory metastatic penile squamous cell carcinoma with extreme durable response to Pembrolizumab. Front Oncol. 2020;10:615298.
28. Hahn AW, Chahoud J, Campbell MT, Karp DD, Wang J, Stephen B, et al. Pembrolizumab for advanced penile cancer: a case series from a phase II basket trial. Investig New Drugs. 2021;
29. McGregor BA, Campbell MT, Xie W, Farah S, Bilen MA, Sonpavde G, et al. Phase II study of nivolumab and ipilimumab for advanced rare genitourinary cancers. J Clin Oncol. 2020;38(15_suppl):5018.

Part IV
Novel Therapeutic Approaches

Chapter 12
Overview of Insightful Systemic Approaches

Savan Shah, Malek Saad, and Jad Chahoud

Introduction

Having discussed the role of systemic therapies in the neoadjuvant, adjuvant, and metastatic settings in the previous chapters, we now turn our attention to novel systemic approaches to penile squamous cell carcinoma (PSCC). The prognosis for patients with advanced platinum refractory PSCC is dismal with a survival rate of less than 5 months, highlighting the need for the development of novel therapeutics. Genomic studies have provided substantial knowledge regarding the genetic and molecular landscape for PSCC; therefore, targeted therapies against genomic alterations are needed but we still have little clinical data with targeted therapies. One area of strong interest is human papilloma virus (HPV)-directed therapy. Up to 50% of PSCC tumors harbor HPV DNA, making HPV-directed therapies a robust area of therapeutic interest [1]. On another note, more than half of PSCC tumors show strong programmed ligand-death 1 (PD-L1) expression, which makes PSCC tumors possibly strong candidates for immunotherapy trials that will be discussed in this chapter.

S. Shah
University of South Florida Morsani College of Medicine at H. Lee Moffitt Cancer Center, Tampa, FL, USA
e-mail: Savan.Shah@moffitt.org

M. Saad
Lebanese American University, Beirut, Lebanon
e-mail: malek.saad@lau.edu

J. Chahoud (✉)
Department of GU Oncology H. Lee Moffit Cancer Center, Tampa, FL, USA

Department of Medicine, University of South Florida, Tampa, FL, USA
e-mail: Jad.Chahoud@moffitt.org

© The Author(s), under exclusive license to Springer Nature Switzerland AG 2021
P. E. Spiess, A. Necchi (eds.), *Penile Carcinoma*,
https://doi.org/10.1007/978-3-030-82060-2_12

Targeted

Molecular Landscape of Penile Squamous Cell Carcinoma

Given the rarity of PSCC, the full understanding of the pathogenesis and progression of PSCC is still being developed. As previously mentioned, in a proportion of patients, HPV DNA integrates into the host genome. This leads to overexpression of E6 and E7, which may lead to inactivation of p53 and RB1 and upregulation of telomerase [2]. However, there is active research being done to expand upon our understanding of the mutational signatures of PSCC. Whole exome sequencing of PSCC revealed that PSCC is most similar to head and neck squamous cell carcinoma (HNSC) with significant enrichment for the NOTCH pathway (70.6%) [3–6]. Feber and colleagues were able to differentiate HPV status in PSCC, by identifying an HPV-associated APOBEC mutational signature and NpCpG signature in HPV-negative disease [4]. Further sequencing by Chahoud et al. identified similar signatures with MP1 APOBEC and MP2 DNA mismatch repair and microsatellite instability [3]. In particular, MP1 enrichment was positively correlated with increased tumor burden and significantly worse survival [3, 5]. Other commonly affected pathways included Hippo and RTK-RAS and p53/cell cycle pathways. Enrichment of PIK3CA and CDKN2A were significantly enriched in specific protein loci in sequencing done by Chahoud and colleagues, suggesting they may be driver mutations. In yet another study using targeted sequencing, McDaniel et al. reported amplifications of MYC and CCND1 genes and association with poor outcomes [6]. Regarding PSCC in particular, a few studies have been made that explored the association of driver and passenger genes alterations with carcinogenesis in PSCC.

Finding new personalized targeted therapy for patients with PSCC is difficult due to the limited research around the molecular drivers of PSCC. Targeted therapy has much potential when it comes to improving the overall outcome of patients with PSCC [7]. TP53, CDKN2A, NOTCH1, and PIK3CA were identified recurrent mutations using profiling methods in patients with PSCC [8–10]. However, it is relevant to note that these studies had many limitations, of which are the sample size, number of HPV cases, and variability in molecular testing methods. New studies have proven that 40% of patients with metastatic PSCC can have a potential-targeted therapy opportunity [7]. This includes mutations in MTOR pathway (11%), DNA repair pathway (BRCA2 and ATM GA, in 14%), and tyrosine kinase (EGFR GA in 6%; FGFR3 and ERBB2 GA each in 4%). A study of whole exome sequencing analysis in PSCC found the most common mutations, which were: TP53 (35%), NOTCH1 (35%), CDKN2A (23%), PIK3CA (21%), and DDR genes (20%) [9].

Epidermal Growth Factor Receptor (EGFR) Inhibitor

Epidermal growth factor receptor (EGFR) is significantly expressed by PSCC tumors and metastases and can be detected by immunohistochemistry [11]. But EGFR mutations that can be targeted are not usually found through molecular testing. While anti-EGFR therapy might appear as a potential treatment due to high levels of expression of EGFR detected by IHC, it is worth noting that multiple case reports and retrospective series show minimal clinical value [12]. The HER/PTEN/Akt pathway is also mutated in PSCC and can be used in targeted therapy with the available treatment options [13]. HER3, HER4, and EGFR expressions were shown to be correlated with PSCC, signifying that targeting HER receptors might be of good use [14].

Dacomintinib has been newly approved as a treatment for patients with metastatic non-small cell lung cancer (NSCLC) with EGFR exon 19 deletion or exon 21 L58R substitution mutations [15]. A new phase II study makes use of the second-generation pan HER tyrosine kinase inhibitor Dacomintinib in 28 chemotherapy-naïve patients with locally advanced or metastatic PSCC [16]. Dacomintinib had an ORR of 32.1% with median PFS of 4.1 months and OS of 13.7 months. The treatment resulted in relatively well-tolerated side effects with only 10% grade 3–4 skin rash as the major toxicity. The trial included patients without taking into account their mutational status. Interestingly, when analyzing the study's translational results, patient selection proved necessary in choosing targeted therapies. Dacomintinib was found to be clinically beneficial when dealing with patients that have mutations in downstream effectors of HER receptors, as well as with TERT mutations. This potentially can be a possible therapeutic option for patients that relapsed from first-line chemotherapy options when clinical trials are not available.

NOTCH: Phosophoinositide 3-Kinase (PI3K) Inhibitors

One study showed that enrichment of the NOTCH signaling pathway was implicated in more than half of PSCC samples while others have shown an enrichment at lower rates, with the limitation of sequencing technique and analysis [3]. However, given its similarity to head and neck, clinical developments from the larger HNSC cohorts could expedite the translation to the less common PSCC [3]. The loss of function mutation of NOTCH1 was initially thought to be non-targetable. But we now know from HNSC, there is therapeutic vulnerability with NOTCH1 loss of function mutations to PI3K/mTOR inhibition [17]. Indeed PI3Ka-specific inhibitors have been used to treat patients with advanced breast cancer. The NOTCH1 pathway remains a potent target for PSCC clinical trials exploration.

DNA Damage Repair (DDR) Genes: Poly Adenosine Diphosphate-Ribose Polymerase (PARP) Inhibitors

Mutations in DNA Damage Repair (DDR) genes have been found in up to 20% of PSCC samples [9]. DDR gene mutations are frequently associated with response to ADP ribose polymerase (PARP) inhibitors and platinum therapy. The DDR pathway is important in tumor biology, allowing cancer cells a mechanism to resist damage by chemotherapy and radiotherapy [18]. Given the lack of knowledge of DDR genes in PSCC, one study identified 26 pathogenic or likely pathogenic variants in DDR genes in 23.5% of patients studied [3]. Given the role of platinum therapy in penile cancer, PARP inhibitors remain a potent investigational therapeutic option for PSCC [3].

Immune Therapy and Its Implications

Background

The revolutionary discovery of immune checkpoint inhibitors (PD1/PD-L1 and CTLA-4) and their use in combination with monoclonal antibodies shows much promise in the management of PSCC. Currently, there are many advances in immunotherapy, coupled with excellent therapeutic results, which has led to more detailed studies concerning the feasibility of immunotherapy in PSCC.

Immune Infiltration Patterns (CD8, FOXP3 T Regs)

Tumor infiltrating lymphocytes (TILs) have been investigated for their role in being the trigger for the host immune response to a number of cancers, as well as being involved in immunoediting and immune escape [19]. $CD3^+/CD4^+$ T cells, $CD3^+/CD8^+$ T cells, and $CD3^+/CD4^+/FOXP3^+$ T_{reg} cells after further investigation seem to comprise the population of TILs [20, 21]. The ratio of T_{regs} to $CD4^+$ T ($\%T_{reg}$) has shown a positive association with shorter survival, while tumor infiltrating $CD4^+$ $T^{high}/CD8^+$ $T^{high}/\%T_{reg}^{low}$ independently demonstrated longer overall survival. As proven by the IMvigor210 study, as the presence of $CD8^+$ cells increase within the cancer, a favorable response can be achieved by combining it with atezolizumab [22]. Therefore, higher levels of $CD8^+$ T cells are associated with a favorable prognosis in PSCC.

A recent study examined and characterized 54 PSCC patients' immune microenvironment using immunohistochemistry with immune markers: CD3, CD8, CD68, PD-1, PD-L1, pancytokeratin, and DAPI [23]. This cohort study analyzed the effect of depleting cytotoxic T cell population subtype ($CD3^+/CD8^+/PD-1^+$), indicating that high densities of antigen experienced T cells that are stromal cytotoxic, and which show immune exclusion, were notably correlated with worse median OS (27 vs 102 months p = 0.05). In addition, Ottenhof et al. in 2018 demonstrated that low stromal $CD8^+$ T cell was linked to lymph node metastasis [24]. Finally, Vassallo et al. in 2015 showed that patients suffering from PSCC that are characterized by high presence of tumor infiltrating $FOXP3^+$ T_{reg} cells had a worse disease-free survival probability (HR 2.50, $p = 0.02$) [25].

Programmed Death-Ligand 1 (PD-L1) Expression

Programmed death ligand 1 (PD-L1) has been identified in 40–60% of PSCCs and mainly high-risk HPV-negative tumors. Increased expression of PD-L1 by either cancers or the host immune cells—specifically tumor associated macrophages (TAMs)—has been associated with poor prognosis and lower numbers of TILs. Almost two thirds of primary PSCCs are PD-L1 positive, with PD-L1 positivity indicated by more than 5% expression.

Udager et al. showed that PD-L1 expression in the primary tumor had a notable correlation with lymph node metastasis (LNM, $p = 0.024$) and shorter cancer-specific survival (CSS, $p = 0.0\,11$) using immunohistochemistry on 37 PSCC cases [26]. In addition, Ottenhof et al. demonstrated in a multivariable study of 213 PSCC patients that only diffuse PD-L1 expression in cancer cells was a notable predictor of lymph node metastasis with OR of 2.81 (p-value = 0.05) [27]. Also, a negative status of high-risk human papilloma virus (hrHPV) and diffuse PD-L1 expression in the cancer field were notably associated with an unfavorable disease-specific survival with an HR of 9.73 (p-value <0.01) and HR of 2.81 (p-value = 0.03), respectively.

Trafalis et al. in 2018 demonstrated a partial response to an anti PD-1 monoclonal antibody nivolumab in a patient with advanced hrHPV-negative PSCC refractory to chemotherapy and radiation therapy [28]. The study showed more than 80% reduction in cancer volume after eight cycles of nivolumab. Adding to that, the histology of the patient pretreatment showed more than 5 percent expression of PD-L1 while the histology of the remaining cancerous cells post treatment showed attenuation of PD-L1 expression with notable augmentation of PD-L1 expression on immune cellular elements that surround cancer cells, which is suggestive of the use of combination therapy with an anti-PD-1/PD-L1 agent.

One phase II trial investigating the use of single agent pembrolizumab in rare cancers, including PSCC, showed that single-agent pembrolizumab was well tolerated as salvage therapy in a small cohort of patients with unresectable, locally advanced or metastatic penile SCC. In the small case series, pembrolizumab produced an objective response in an MSI-H tumor, but it did not control disease in two patients with MSS penile SCC [29, 30].

Additional studies have also investigated the role of combined immune checkpoint blockers (ICB). One preclinical study showed that using celecoxib or cabozantinib in addition to a ICB resulted in a synergistic effect leading to the eradication of most tumor nodules [31]. One phase I study examined the safety and efficacy of cabozantinib plus nivolumab with or without Ipilumumab in a variety of metastatic and advanced genitourinary cancers and included three patients with PSCC. Significantly, grade 3 or 4 immune-related side effects occurred in 87% of patients receiving all three therapies and in 75% receiving cabozantinib and nivolumab. Clinical activity showed one patient with partial response and two with stable disease [32]. Finally, a similar phase I study showed the effect of combined nivolumab and ipilumumab in advanced GU cancers. Within this study, there were five PSCC patients with evaluable response. Of those two had stable disease and three had progressive disease [33].

Finally, for the first time, the FDA granted tumor agnostic approval for the use of pembrolizumab in patients with relapsed advanced solid cancers, DNA mismatch repair-deficient tumors, or microsatellite instability-high (MSI-H) tumors based on several recent studies, including KEYNOTE-158. One study reported an ORR of 71% across several tumor types. However, a study assessing the prevalence of MSI-H in PSCC has shown low rates of MSI-H PSCC, which would limit the clinical use of pembrolizumab based on the abovementioned FDA approval [9]. Nevertheless, other predictive markers of response to checkpoint inhibitors exist, similar to the tumor mutational burden of ≥ 10 mutations per Mb, as it was shown in lung cancer [34]. One group reported that 21% of PSCC specimens were found to have ≥ 10 mutations per Mb [10]. Therefore, a continuing rationale exists for drug development with immune checkpoint blockade to treat patients with an aggressive cancer and dismal survival.

Macrophage Infiltration Patterns

TAMs have an essential role in the cancer's microenvironment through regulating immunotolerance, amplifying cancer cell mobility, and enhancing angiogenesis. VEGF is shown to be correlated with TAMs and TGF-B, and the expression of VEGF has been proven to be an independent prognostic factor for metastatic progression in PSCC [35]. Additionally, TAMs have been proven to be part of the establishment of pre-metastatic niches, which may be involved in a cancer survival mechanism against systemic chemotherapy [36]. New studies show that IL-6/JAK/STAT3 signaling pathway can be a therapeutic target to suppress cancer growth and activate the antitumor immune response [37]. However, it is worth mentioning that in a couple of small phase II clinical trials, the use of anti-IL-6 antibody in metastatic castration-resistant prostate cancer and in advanced solid tumors did not demonstrate clinical benefit [38, 39].

In PSCC, high concentrations of CD68$^+$ TAMs were correlated with markedly improved cancer-specific survival (CSS) ($p = 0.04$), overall survival (OS) ($p = 0.02$), and lower risk of regional recurrence ($p = 0.04$). Another PSCC group found increased intra-tumoral CD163$^+$ which corresponds with LNM [20].

HPV-Directed Therapies

There is an interest in the correlation of HPV and PSCC, as it is an area of active research for immunotherapy augmentation. Differences in sampling, viral molecular testing, and population studied can lead to variation in the prevalence and incidence reported of HPV. However, a systematic review of 1266 invasive PSCC patients showed that in North America up to 48.7% of PSCCs harbor HPV DNA [1]. High-risk HPV (hrHPV), 16 and 18 subtypes specifically, composed a significant majority of HPV-positive PSCC cases: 30.8% and 6.6%, respectively [1]. Stratified by HPV status, 213 PSCC patients with hrHPV negativity were associated substantially with poor disease-specific survival (HR 9.7, $p < 0.01$). HPV positivity in PSCC has repeatedly shown better outcomes in survival, which can be associated to elevated production of neo-antigens.

Numerous HPV targeting therapies have been and are currently being studied. In particular, a phase I/II investigated autologous genetically engineered T-cells expressing a T-cell receptor directed against HPV16 E6 in combination with a conditioning regimen and systemic aldesleukin. Doran and colleagues enrolled 12 patients with metastatic HPV16-positive cancer from any primary tumor site who had received prior platinum-based therapy to receive the autologous engineered T-cells [40]. Two patients in the highest dose cohort experienced objective tumor responses. This landmark study showed the feasibility and potential clinical activity of this novel HPV-directed approach.

Conclusions

PSCC is a rare cancer of increasing prevalence due to many risk factors and improved epidemiological studies worldwide. Though localized PSCC has been treated successfully surgically, patients that develop advanced PSCC with metastatic potential usually have dismal prognosis when the disease is refractory to cisplatin-based therapy. Additionally, the conventional use of chemotherapy and radiation does not make the prognosis any better, rendering exploring new treatment options essential. Subsequently, these factors led to many new studies with high potential, mainly targeted therapy, immune therapy, and HPV therapeutic and preventative-based therapies.

References

1. Dillner J, Von Krogh G, Horenblas S, Meijer CJLM. Etiology of squamous cell carcinoma of the penis. Scand J Urol Nephrol Suppl. 2000; https://doi.org/10.1080/00365590050509913.
2. Kidd LC, Chaing S, Chipollini J, Giuliano AR, Spiess PE, Sharma P. Relationship between human papillomavirus and penile cancer-implications for prevention and treatment. Transl Androl Urol. 2017;6:791–802.
3. Chahoud J, Gleber-Netto FO, McCormick BZ, et al. Whole exome sequencing in penile squamous cell carcinoma uncovers novel prognostic categorization and drug targets similar to head and neck squamous cell carcinoma. Clin Cancer Res. 2021; https://doi.org/10.1158/1078-0432.ccr-20-4004.
4. McGregor BA, Sonpavde GP. New insights into the molecular profile of penile squamous cell carcinoma. Clin Cancer Res. 2021;27:2375–7.

5. Feber A, Worth DC, Chakravarthy A, et al. CSN1 somatic mutations in penile squamous cell carcinoma. Cancer Res. 2016;76:4720–7.

6. McDaniel AS, Hovelson DH, Cani AK, et al. Genomic profiling of penile squamous cell carcinoma reveals new opportunities for targeted therapy. Cancer Res. 2015;75:5219–27.

7. Chahoud J, Pickering CR, Pettaway CA. Genetics and penile cancer: recent developments and implications. Curr Opin Urol. 2019; https://doi.org/10.1097/MOU.0000000000000640.

8. Ali SM, Pal SK, Wang K, et al. Comprehensive genomic profiling of advanced penile carcinoma suggests a high frequency of clinically relevant genomic alterations. Oncologist. 2016; https://doi.org/10.1634/theoncologist.2015-0241.

9. Jacob JM, Ferry EK, Gay LM, et al. Comparative genomic profiling of refractory and metastatic penile and nonpenile cutaneous squamous cell carcinoma: implications for selection of systemic therapy. J Urol. 2019; https://doi.org/10.1016/j.juro.2018.09.056.

10. Chahoud J, McCormick BZ, Netto F, Rao P, Pickering CR, Pettaway CA. Penile squamous cell carcinoma is genomically similar to other HPV-driven tumors. J Clin Oncol. 2019; https://doi.org/10.1200/jco.2019.37.7_suppl.505.

11. Gu W, Zhu Y, Ye D. Beyond chemotherapy for advanced disease - the role of EGFR and PD-1 inhibitors. Transl Androl Urol. 2017;6:848–54.

12. Northrup BE, Jokerst CE, Grubb RL, Menias CO, Khanna G, Siegel CL. Hereditary renal tumor syndromes: imaging findings and management strategies. Am J Roentgenol. 2012; https://doi.org/10.2214/AJR.12.9079.

13. Stankiewicz E, Prowse DM, Ng M, et al. Alternative HER/PTEN/Akt pathway activation in HPV positive and negative penile carcinomas. PLoS One. 2011;6:e17517.

14. Hsieh AC, Moasser MM. Targeting HER proteins in cancer therapy and the role of the nontarget HER3. Br J Cancer. 2007;97:453–7.

15. Wu YL, Cheng Y, Zhou X, et al. Dacomitinib versus gefitinib as first-line treatment for patients with EGFR-mutation-positive non-small-cell lung cancer (ARCHER 1050): a randomised, open-label, phase 3 trial. Lancet Oncol. 2017; https://doi.org/10.1016/S1470-2045(17)30608-3.

16. Necchi A, Lo Vullo S, Perrone F, et al. First-line therapy with dacomitinib, an orally available pan-HER tyrosine kinase inhibitor, for locally advanced or metastatic penile squamous cell carcinoma: results of an open-label, single-arm, single-centre, phase 2 study. BJU Int. 2018;121:348–56.

17. Sambandam V, Frederick MJ, Shen L, et al. PDK1 mediates Notch1-mutated head and neck squamous carcinoma vulnerability to therapeutic PI3K/mTOR inhibition. Clin Cancer Res. 2019; https://doi.org/10.1158/1078-0432.CCR-18-3276.

18. O'Connor MJ. Targeting the DNA damage response in cancer. Mol Cell. 2015; https://doi.org/10.1016/j.molcel.2015.10.040.

19. Gooden MJM, De Bock GH, Leffers N, Daemen T, Nijman HW. The prognostic influence of tumour-infiltrating lymphocytes in cancer: a systematic review with meta-analysis. Br J Cancer. 2011; https://doi.org/10.1038/bjc.2011.189.

20. de Vries HM, Ottenhof SR, Horenblas S, van der Heijden MS, Jordanova ES. Defining the tumor microenvironment of penile cancer by means of the cancer Immunogram. Eur Urol Focus. 2019; https://doi.org/10.1016/j.euf.2019.02.019.

21. Ino Y, Yamazaki-Itoh R, Shimada K, Iwasaki M, Kosuge T, Kanai Y, Hiraoka N. Immune cell infiltration as an indicator of the immune microenvironment of pancreatic cancer. Br J Cancer. 2013; https://doi.org/10.1038/bjc.2013.32.

22. Necchi A, Joseph RW, Loriot Y, et al. Atezolizumab in platinum-treated locally advanced or metastatic urothelial carcinoma: post-progression outcomes from the phase II IMvigor210 study. Ann Oncol. 2017; https://doi.org/10.1093/annonc/mdx518.

23. Chahoud J, Netto F, Lazcano Segura R, Parra Cuentas ER, Lu X, Rao P, Wistuba II, Pickering CR, Pettaway CA. Tumor immune microenvironment alterations in penile squamous cell carcinoma using multiplex immunofluorescence and image analysis approaches. J Clin Oncol. 2020; https://doi.org/10.1200/jco.2020.38.6_suppl.4.

24. Ottenhof SR, Djajadiningrat RS, Thygesen HH, Jakobs PJ, Józwiak K, Heeren AM, de Jong J, Sanders J, Horenblas S, Jordanova ES. The prognostic value of immune factors in the tumor microenvironment of penile squamous cell carcinoma. Front Immunol. 2018; https://doi.org/10.3389/fimmu.2018.01253.
25. Vassallo J, Rodrigues AFF, Campos AHJFM, et al. Pathologic and imunohistochemical characterization of tumoral inflammatory cell infiltrate in invasive penile squamous cell carcinomas: fox-P3 expression is an independent predictor of recurrence. Tumor Biol. 2015; https://doi.org/10.1007/s13277-014-2864-2.
26. Udager AM, Liu TY, Skala SL, et al. Frequent PD-L1 expression in primary and metastatic penile squamous cell carcinoma: potential opportunities for immunotherapeutic approaches. Ann Oncol. 2016; https://doi.org/10.1093/annonc/mdw216.
27. Ottenhof SR, Djajadiningrat RS, de Jong J, Thygesen HH, Horenblas S, Jordanova ES. Expression of programmed death ligand 1 in penile cancer is of prognostic value and associated with HPV status. J Urol. 2017; https://doi.org/10.1016/j.juro.2016.09.088.
28. Trafalis DT, Alifieris CE, Kalantzis A, Verigos KE, Vergadis C, Sauvage S. Evidence for efficacy of treatment with the anti-PD-1 Mab Nivolumab in radiation and Multichemorefractory advanced penile squamous cell carcinoma. J Immunother. 2018; https://doi.org/10.1097/CJI.0000000000000221.
29. Hahn AW, Chahoud J, Campbell MT, Karp DD, Wang J, Stephen B, Tu SM, Pettaway CA, Naing A. Pembrolizumab for advanced penile cancer: a case series from a phase II basket trial. Investig New Drugs. 2021; https://doi.org/10.1007/s10637-021-01100-x.
30. Naing A, Meric-Bernstam F, Stephen B, et al. Phase 2 study of pembrolizumab in patients with advanced rare cancers. J Immunother Cancer. 2020; https://doi.org/10.1136/jitc-2019-000347.
31. Huang T, Cheng X, Chahoud J, et al. Effective combinatorial immunotherapy for penile squamous cell carcinoma. Nat Commun. 2020; https://doi.org/10.1038/s41467-020-15980-9.
32. Apolo AB, Nadal R, Girardi DM, et al. Phase I study of Cabozantinib and Nivolumab alone or with Ipilimumab for advanced or metastatic urothelial carcinoma and other genitourinary tumors. J Clin Oncol. 2020; https://doi.org/10.1200/JCO.20.01652.
33. McGregor BA, Campbell MT, Xie W, et al. Phase II study of nivolumab and ipilimumab for advanced rare genitourinary cancers. J Clin Oncol. 2020; https://doi.org/10.1200/jco.2020.38.15_suppl.5018.
34. Hellmann MD, Ciuleanu T-E, Pluzanski A, et al. Nivolumab plus Ipilimumab in lung cancer with a high tumor mutational burden. N Engl J Med. 2018; https://doi.org/10.1056/nejmoa1801946.
35. De Paula AAP, Motta ED, Alencar RDC, Saddi VA, Da Silva RC, Caixeta GN, Almeida Netto JC, Carneiro MADS. The impact of cyclooxygenase-2 and vascular endothelial growth factor C immunoexpression on the prognosis of penile carcinoma. J Urol. 2012; https://doi.org/10.1016/j.juro.2011.09.027.
36. Valastyan S, Weinberg RA. Tumor metastasis: molecular insights and evolving paradigms. Cell. 2011; https://doi.org/10.1016/j.cell.2011.09.024.
37. Kitamura H, Ohno Y, Toyoshima Y, Ohtake J, Homma S, Kawamura H, Takahashi N, Taketomi A. Interleukin-6/STAT3 signaling as a promising target to improve the efficacy of cancer immunotherapy. Cancer Sci. 2017; https://doi.org/10.1111/cas.13332.
38. Fizazi K, De Bono JS, Flechon A, et al. Randomised phase II study of siltuximab (CNTO 328), an anti-IL-6 monoclonal antibody, in combination with mitoxantrone/prednisone versus mitoxantrone/prednisone alone in metastatic castration-resistant prostate cancer. Eur J Cancer. 2012; https://doi.org/10.1016/j.ejca.2011.10.014.
39. Angevin E, Tabernero J, Elez E, et al. A phase I/II, multiple-dose, dose-escalation study of siltuximab, an anti-interleukin-6 monoclonal antibody, in patients with advanced solid tumors. Clin Cancer Res. 2014; https://doi.org/10.1158/1078-0432.CCR-13-2200.
40. Doran SL, Stevanović S, Adhikary S, et al. T-cell receptor gene therapy for human papillomavirus-associated epithelial cancers: a first-in-human, phase I/II study. J Clin Oncol. 2019;37:2759–68.

Chapter 13
Clinical Trials Corner

Andrea Necchi and Philippe E. Spiess

Latest Evidences and Future Role of Immune-Checkpoint Inhibition in Advanced Penile Carcinoma

Checkpoint inhibitors have revolutionized the treatment paradigms of several solid tumors, mainly of those tumors with certain molecular characteristics added to the immunohistochemical expression of programmed death-1/ligand-1 (PD-1/PD-L1) biomarker.

By analyzing the database of Foundation Medicine Inc., including a total of 230 cases from patients with clinically advanced PSCC, the authors have reported the most recent update on the frequency of biomarkers potentially associated with activity of anti-PD-1/PD-L1 agents [1]. In this cohort, the proportion of cases revealing a tumor mutational burden (TMB) higher than 10 mutations/Mb was 15%, and those showing a PD-L1 expression on tumor cells or immune cells equal or higher than 50% was 34%. Interestingly, these proportions do not seem to be significantly different between the cohorts of human papillomavirus (HPV)-positive or negative PSCC [2]. Conversely, the proportion of PSCC showing a microsatellite instability-high feature is confirmed to be very low (1%).

Initial experiences with checkpoint inhibition in patients with PSCC who were refractory to standard therapies have been reported in a few case reports, with

A. Necchi (✉)
Vita-Salute San Raffaele University, IRCCS San Raffaele Hospital and Scientific Institute, Milan, Italy
e-mail: andrea.necchi@istitutotumori.mi.it

P. E. Spiess
Department of Genito-Urinary Oncology, Department of Tumor Biology, H. Lee Moffitt Cancer Center and Research Institute, Tampa, FL, USA
e-mail: Philippe.Spiess@moffitt.org

contrasting evidence of activity [3, 4]. Certainly, the role of immunotherapy and, in particular, selecting the optimal therapeutic strategy between single-agent and combinatorial therapy is still hard based on the available data. Overall, it seems that using immunotherapy-based compounds alone, either as single agents or immune combinations, would be hard to achieve significant tumor volume reduction, at least to envision a future role of such therapies in earlier, perioperative stages.

The ongoing studies using immune-checkpoint inhibitors offered today to patients with PSCC are presented in Table 13.1.

Among the ongoing studies, one of the largest collaborative efforts is represented by the "Orpheus" study (NCT042319819), testing the activity of a novel anti-PD-1 compound, INCMGA00012. This is a multicenter, open-label, single-arm phase 2 study running in Europe, including patients with locally advanced or metastatic PSCC who are chemo-naive or have already received one course of standard cisplatin-based chemotherapy. The primary endpoint of the study is the objective response rate, according to the Response Evaluation Criteria in Solid Tumors (RECIST), version 1.1. A total number of 18 patients is planned to be accrued within Q2, 2021. Another intriguing study is the French "Pulse" trial (NCT03774901) testing the efficacy of the anti-PD-L1 antibody avelumab in the setting of maintenance therapy after first-line chemotherapy, which has not been addressed so far by previous studies.

Among the studies whose data have been already reported, we also have results from combination therapies like the combination of nivolumab and cabozantinib, with or without ipilimumab, that was tested in a phase 1 basket trial by the National Cancer Institute (NCI) in the United States [5]. Three patients with advanced PSCC have been included in this study. These patients benefited from either a partial response (N = 1) or a stable disease (N = 2) from treatment.

The combination of ipilimumab and nivolumab was also tested in another basket study including patients with rare genitourinary malignancies [6]. In this study, six patients with clinically advanced PSSCC received treatment, but only two of them benefited with a minimal response/stable disease from treatment.

Another intriguing strategy using immunotherapy that is being tested in clinical trials like the "Pericles" study (NCT03686332) is represented by its combination with radical radiotherapy (RT). Harnessing the systemic effect of local RT is an intriguing concept that relies on noteworthy observations from preclinical studies and very early clinical data [7]. For example, focal RT enhanced systemic responses to anti-CTLA-4 antibodies in preclinical and clinical studies in melanoma and non-small-cell lung cancers, and RT promoted the activation of anti-tumor T-cells, an effect dependent on type I interferon-γ induction in the irradiated tumors.

Further, there is considerable data, across tumor types, that there is synergy between RT and immunotherapy. This forms the basis for considering immune RT strategies utilizing immune checkpoint inhibitors as part of the systemic therapy regimen in patients with inguinal lymph node involvement from PSCC.

Finally, the latest developments of immunotherapy strategies in PSCC are now focusing on the use of cellular therapies and therapeutic vaccines, directed against HPV antigens, currently being offered to patients within phase 1 studies, as detailed

Table 13.1 Ongoing and active clinical trials with novel immunotherapeutic approaches including patients with penile cancers (registered at ClinicalTrial.gov [a])

Trial ID (acronym)	Geographical allocation	Treatment	Experimental drug category	Clinical setting	Planned completion year	Total N (Penile cancer)
NCT03686332 (PERICLES)	The Netherlands	Atezolizumab +/− RT	Anti-PD-L1	First-line	2021	32
NCT04475016	China	TIP+Nimotuzumab & Triprilimab	Anti-EGFR & anti-PD-1	Neoadjuvant	2022	29
NCT04224740	Brazil (LACOG)	Pembrolizumab + platinum/5FU	Anti-PD-1	First-line	2022	33
NCT02817958	France (UNICANCER)	TIP + ILND	CT	Neoadjuvant/adjuvant	2021	37
NCT03391479	Canada (Princess Margaret Hospital)	Avelumab	Anti-PD-L1	First and second line	2021	24
NCT03774901 (pulse)	France	Avelumab	Anti-PD-L1	Maintenance after first line	2022	32
NCT04231981 (ORPHEUS)	International European	INCMGA00012 (retifanlimab)	Anti-PD-1	First and second line	2022	18
NCT04718584	China	LDP	Anti-PD-L1	Salvage therapy	2021	27
NCT02496208	United States (NCI)	Cabozantinib/Nivolumab +/− Ipilimumab	TKI Anti-PD-L1 Anti-CTLA4	Salvage therapy	2021	n.a.
NCT04357873 (PEVOsq)	France (UNICANCER)	Pembrolizumab + vorinostat	Anti-PD-L1 HDAC inhibitor	Salvage therapy	2023	n.a.
NCT02721732	United States (MDACC)	Pembrolizumab	Anti-PD-1	Salvage therapy	2021	n.a.
NCT03333616	United States (DFCI)	Nivolumab + Ipilimumab	Anti-PD-1 Anti-CTLA4	First and second line	2021	n.a.
NCT04272034	International Incyte	INCB099318	Anti-PD-1	Salvage therapy	2022	n.a.

(continued)

Table 13.1 (continued)

Trial ID (acronym)	Geographical allocation	Treatment	Experimental drug category	Clinical setting	Planned completion year	Total N (Penile cancer)
NCT02834013	United States NCI	Nivolumab + Ipilimumab	Anti-PD-1 Anti-CTLA4	Salvage therapy	2021	n.a.
HPV-directed strategies						
NCT02858310	United States (NCI)	TCR targeting HPV-16 E7 (E7 TCR) + aldesleukin	Anti-HPV engineered T-cells; Human recombinant interleukin-2	Salvage therapy	2026	n.a.
NCT02379520	United States (Baylor College of Medicine)	HPV specific T cells + nivolumab + CT	Anti-HPV vaccine Anti-PD-1	Salvage therapy	2021	n.a.
NCT03439085	Unites States (MDACC)	INO-3112 and durvalumab	Anti-HPV vaccine Anti-PD-L1	Salvage therapy	2021	n.a.
NCT04180215	United States (Hookipa Biotech GmbH)	HB-201 single vector therapy and HB-201 & HB-202 two-vector therapy	Viral vector therapy	Salvage therapy	2022	n.a.

Abbreviations: CT chemotherapy, *CTLA4* Cytotoxic T-Lymphocyte Antigen 4, *EGFR* epidermal growth-factor receptor, *FU* fluorouracil, *HDAC* histone deacetylase, *HPV* human papillomavirus, *PD-L1* programmed cell-death-ligand-1, *RT* radiotherapy, *TIP* paclitaxel, ifosfamide, cisplatin
[a] Accessed on June first, 2021

in Table 13.1. HPV-related oncoproteins are, in fact, a potential source of immuno-genic neoantigens. HB-201 and HB-202 are replicating live-attenuated vectors based on lymphocytic choriomeningitis virus and Pichinde virus, respectively, which express the same non-oncogenic HPV16 E7E6 fusion protein to induce tumor-specific T-cell responses. The initial results of the first-in-human phase 1/2 study of HB-201 monotherapy and HB-201 & HB-202 alternating 2-vector therapy have been recently presented by Ho and colleagues (NCT04180215) [8]. In a total of 25 patients with HPV-related malignancies refractory to standard treatments, ini-tial signals of antitumor activity have been reported with a well-tolerated safety profile.

Putative Non-Immunotherapy-Based Strategies and Future Directions

Emerging evidence is supporting the concept of jointly developing new agents in penile cancer and head and neck SCC due to the significant amount of potentially overlapping genomic alterations as recently highlighted [1].

In fact, PSCC had genomic features more similar to head and neck SCC than other SCC of the pelvic region (e.g., urethral SCC), including slightly increased cell-cycle perturbation, HPV infection, and in particular NOTCH signaling pathway alterations.

Genomic alterations in *NOTCH1* have been reported in about 25% of cases [9] with clinically advanced penile cancer, with a select enrichment in tumors associ-ated with HPV infection. *NOTCH1* mutations have now emerged both as targets of novel anti-NOTCH pathway drugs and potential immune-checkpoint inhibi-tors resistance biomarkers [10–12]. As an example, in patients with colorectal cancer, the modulation of NOTCH signaling promoted the cytotoxicity of CD8+ T-cells by decreasing PD-1 expression, and also promoted the production of interferon-γ.

More than 70 clinical trials using NOTCH inhibitors are now registered on ClinicalTrials.gov, and the first-ever phase III trial of a NOTCH gamma secretase inhibitor, nirogacestat, is currently ongoing (NCT03785964).

Other rarer but potentially targetable genomic alterations identified in PSCC included NF1mutations (7%), PTEN (4%), tyrosine kinase receptors gene altera-tions (*EGFR* 6%, *FGFR3* 4%, *ERBB2* 4%), and DNA repair pathway alterations (*BRCA2* 7%, *ATM* 7%) [1, 2, 13].

From all these premises, it is rather clear that the future of advanced PSCC treat-ment should rely on the possibility of including these patients in basket studies with early new drugs. In general, developing newer agents specifically addressed to these tumors should be discouraged, as most of the opportunities that may come from clinical studies in the field are more related to the optimization of already available strategies rather than the identification of newer ones. The InPACT study (NCT02305654) best exemplifies this paradigm.

References

1. Spiess PE, Mata DA, Bratslavsky G, et al. Clinically advanced penile (pSCC) and male urethral (uSCC) squamous cell carcinoma: a comparative genomic profiling (CGP) study. J Clin Oncol. 2021;39(suppl 6); abstr 2.
2. Bandini M. Ross JS, Zhu Y, et al. Association between human papillomavirus infection and outcome of perioperative nodal radiotherapy for penile carcinoma. Eur Urol Oncol. 2020;S2588–9311(20)30176-0 (Epub ahead of print).
3. Hahn AW, Chahoud J, Campbell MT, et al. Pembrolizumab for advanced penile cancer: a case series from a phase II basket trial. Invest New Drugs. 2021 Mar 26. https://doi.org/10.1007/s10637-021-01100-x. Online ahead of print.
4. Chahoud J, Skelton WP 4th, Spiess PE, et al. Case report: two cases of chemotherapy refractory metastatic penile squamous cell carcinoma with extreme durable response to Pembrolizumab. Front Oncol. 2020;10:615298.
5. Apolo AB, Nadal R, Girardi DM, et al. Phase I study of Cabozantinib and Nivolumab alone or with Ipilimumab for advanced or metastatic urothelial carcinoma and other genitourinary tumors. J Clin Oncol. 2020;38:3672–84.
6. McGregor BA, Campbell MT, Xie W, et al. Results of a multicenter, phase 2 study of nivolumab and ipilimumab for patients with advanced rare genitourinary malignancies. Cancer. 2021;127:840–9.
7. Formenti SC, Rudqvist NP, Golden E, et al. Radiotherapy induces responses of lung cancer to CTLA-4 blockade. Nat Med. 2018;24:1845–51.
8. Ho AL, Posner MR, Niu J, et al. First report of the safety/tolerability and preliminary antitumor activity of HB-201 and HB-202, an arenavirus-based cancer immunotherapy, in patients with HPV16+ cancers. J Clin Oncol. 2021;39(suppl 15); abstr 2502.
9. Ali SM, Pal SK, Wang K, et al. Comprehensive genomic profiling of advanced penile carcinoma suggests a high frequency of clinically relevant genomic alterations. Oncologist. 2016;21:33–9.
10. Moore G, Annett S, McClements L, et al. Top Notch targeting strategies in cancer: a detailed overview of recent insights and current perspectives. Cell. 2020;9:1503.
11. Yu W, Wang Y, Guo P. Notch signaling pathway dampens tumor-infiltrating CD8+ T cells activity in patients with colorectal carcinoma. Biomed Pharmacother. 2018;97:535–42.
12. Chahoud J, Gleber-Netto FO, McCormick BZ, et al. Whole-exome sequencing in penile squamous cell carcinoma uncovers novel prognostic categorization and drug targets similar to head and neck squamous cell carcinoma. Clin Cancer Res. 2021;27:2560–70.
13. Aydin AM, Chahoud J, Adashek JJ, et al. Understanding genomics and the immune environment of penile cancer to improve therapy. Nat Rev Urol. 2020;17:555–70.

Index

Printed in the United States
by Baker & Taylor Publisher Services